American Food Habits in Historical Perspective

AMERICAN FOOD HABITS IN HISTORICAL PERSPECTIVE

Elaine N. McIntosh, Ph.D., R.D.

PRAEGER

Westport, Connecticut
London

Library of Congress Cataloging-in-Publication Data

McIntosh, Elaine N.
  American food habits in historical perspective / Elaine N.
McIntosh.
    p.   cm.
  Includes bibliographical references and index.
  ISBN 0–275–94601–0 (alk. paper).—ISBN 0–275–95331–9 (pbk.)
    1. Food habits—United States—History.   2. Diet—United States—
History.   3. Nutrition—United States—History.   4. United States—
Social life and customs.   I. Title.
GT2853.U5M39   1995
394.1'2'0973—dc20   95–7550

British Library Cataloguing in Publication Data is available.

Library of Congress Catalog Card Number: 95–7550
ISBN: 0–275–94601–0
       0–275–95331–9 (pbk.)

First published in 1995

Praeger Publishers, 88 Post Road West, Westport, CT 06881
An imprint of Greenwood Publishing Group, Inc.

Printed in the United States of America

The paper used in this book complies with the
Permanent Paper Standard issued by the National
Information Standards Organization (Z39.48–1984).

10 9 8 7 6 5 4 3 2 1

Contents

Illustrations

TABLES

Preface

Food habits are not independent entities. They reflect, and are influenced by, the entire ecological milieu in which they occur. Therefore, the study of food habits calls for an interdisciplinary approach, utilizing both the biological and social sciences, including biology, physiology, history, sociology, psychology, anthropology, and nutrition (as well as the relatively new science of nutritional anthropology).

This book provides a historical overview of the food habits of human beings over time, with special emphasis on American dietary habits from Columbian times through the present (chapters 4, 5, 6, 9, and 10). Food habits are addressed within the context of the relevant events, developments, and circumstances associated with each era.

Chapter 1 introduces the reader to the essentiality of food as a source of nourishment for all living things. The basic concepts of nutrition are explained, and significant milestones in the history of nutrition are presented. Finally, the associations between human evolution and changing nutritional needs and diets of human beings are addressed.

Because sufficient food is pivotal to the existence of society, human beings have devoted much time and effort to obtaining an adequate food supply. Chapter 2 describes the various traditional methods of obtaining food, the characteristics of food-gathering and food-producing societies, the elements of food processing, and the universal foods and food products that have been used by human cultures across time. Such information should be helpful to the reader in developing an awareness of the commonalities among cultures with respect to various food habits and practices. It also should aid the reader in gaining a perspective from which to compare and assess the food habits of various eras, areas, and cultures.

Chapter 3 focuses on early dietary patterns of the ancestors of post-Columbian North Americans, especially with respect to those in Europe and in North America, prior to the landfall of Columbus in the Bahamas in 1492. Aside from its intrinsic interest, this information should provide insight as to the degree of influence these ancestral eating habits may have had on the subsequent dietary patterns of North Americans during the post-Columbian era.

Two chapters—chapter 7, Understanding Food Habits, and chapter 8, Food and Ideology—focus on factors that influence foods habits.

Chapter 9 provides an in-depth characterization of contemporary American food habits. Mainstream cuisine, regional cooking (including "regional phenomena"), and pop food are examined. Important influences on these types of cooking are identified and described. This is an exhaustive subject, about which much more could have been written. The author particularly regrets that space limitations prevented a more extensive treatment of ethnic foods, which add so much interest to the American culinary scene.

Chapter 10 assesses the nutritional adequacy of American diets during various periods from prehistoric times up to the present, using information regarding food habits and food consumption, along with available nutrition-related health statistics. Finally, some predictions regarding the American diet of the future are made.

The interested reader is encouraged to seek more information on selected topics presented in the book, using other sources, beginning with those listed at the end of each chapter, under "For Further Reference."

The author wishes to thank the numerous individuals and organizations who provided pictures for the book: Tom McIntosh, Ph.D.; Nancy Sell, Ph.D.; Neville Public Museum of Brown County; The Wisconsin Historical Society; Library of Congress; National Archives; United States Department of Agriculture, Agricultural Research Service; United States Department of Agriculture, Office of Public Affairs; The B. Maneschewitz Company; General Mills, Inc.; and PET, Inc. The author is most grateful to her husband, Tom McIntosh, for his unfailing support and helpful advice throughout the preparation of the manuscript.

American Food Habits
in Historical Perspective

Humans, Nutrition, and Survival

Humans, like other living things, are physiological beings who require nourishment for the growth and maintenance of their bodies and for other important functions. This nourishment comes from food. Because food is so central to survival, it is not surprising that the hunger drive is so strong.

Historically, people have been obliged to eat whatever foods were available, primarily to appease hunger. Only after this basic drive of hunger was satisfied were people in a position to be selective regarding food choices. Through experience, they learned which foods were conducive to health and well-being and which were dangerous and to be avoided.

NUTRITIONAL SCIENCE

Food contains substances, needed and used by the body, known as nutrients. There are many kinds of foods, and the nutrients they contain differ in kind and amount. The process whereby food is assimilated and used by the body is called nutrition. The study and understanding of this process, on the other hand, is called nutritional science.

Since food always has been a universal need, it is no wonder that it has been the focus of much attention throughout human history. Not only has the procurement of food itself occupied much of man's time; food also has occupied much of man's thoughts. Very early, man became aware of the relationship between adequate food and well-being. Those persons who did

Figure 1.1
Food Is Essential for Life

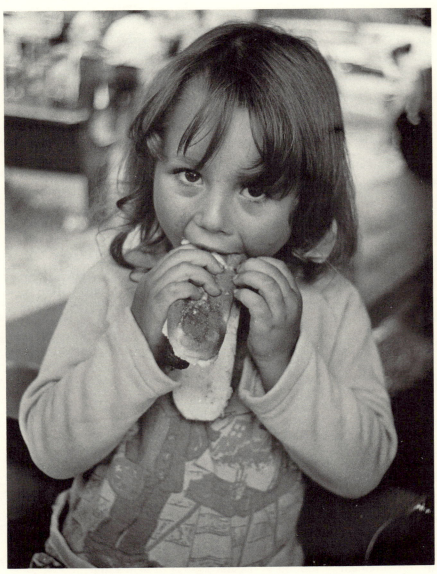

Press Gazette Collection of the Neville Public Museum of Brown County

not have sufficient food starved to death. This awareness has evoked count-less observations regarding the relationship between food and health throughout history. Although many of these observations have been shown to be invalid, others have proved to be surprisingly insightful, withstanding the test of scientific inquiry. Over time, inquiring people the world over, from a wide range of backgrounds, have contributed much to our present knowledge of nutrition. The story of the evolution of nutritional science is a fascinating one, of which only a brief overview can be presented here.

Early History

The story of human nutrition undoubtedly began with the emergence of people and their need for sustenance. Indeed, the importance of food and making proper food choices for early humans can be inferred from the story of Adam and Eve in chapters 2 and 3 of Genesis, the first book of the Holy Bible. Here, God is said to have commanded Adam to eat freely of every tree in the Garden of Eden, except for the fruit from the tree of knowledge.[1]

Information regarding the earliest beliefs regarding nutrition have come from diverse sources, including ancient Babylonian and Egyptian tablets, manuscripts written on scrolls of leather and papyrus, and early Greek and Roman records. The perceptions regarding nutrition of people in later times have been inferred from various sources. They include journals of explorers and voyagers, records of wars and famines, diaries and letters, medical records and scientific writings (Lowenberg, Todhunter, Wilson, Savage, and Lubawski 1979).

The earliest nutrition-related record is that of Ebert's papyrus, an Egyptian medical treatise, dated at 1500 B.C. It included recommendations for eating roast ox liver or the liver of black cock to cure night blindness. It now is known that this condition is caused by a lack of vitamin A and that liver is an especially rich source of this vitamin. Scurvy (now known to be caused by insufficient vitamin C) also is discussed in this ancient document. The earliest record of a nutrition experiment with human subjects, com-paring two diets, is found in the book of Daniel 1:1–15. The experiment was conducted by Nebuchadnezzar, King of Babylon, after taking control of Jerusalem in 607 B.C. Daniel requested that he and his young Jewish associates be excused from eating the king's food and wine, which, custom-arily, were fed the noble youths selected for training as courtiers, and be allowed, instead, to subsist on pulses (peas or other leguminous vegetables). After 10 days, they were better in appearance and fatter in flesh than the youths who had partaken of the king's fare (McCollum 1957:8–9).

During the Classical period, a number of early Greek physicians and

[1]The contents of Genesis and the other books of the Law were kept alive through oral tradition until about 900–1000 B.C., when they began to be written down.

philosophers proposed theories related to food and nutrition, which have been upheld by later scientific investigations. However, true progress in nutrition was impossible without a knowledge of the chemistry of living things (Lusk 1922).

This scientific impasse continued after the Fall of Rome (476 A.D.) through the High Middle Ages (the end of the thirteenth century). During this time, there was little emphasis on learning and scientific endeavor. The energies of Western Europeans were focused on the spread of Christianity and the Crusades (aimed at recapturing the Holy Land).

The Renaissance

With the Renaissance (between the fourteenth and the sixteenth centuries) came a revival of learning that followed a long period of largely clerical studies in both the Middle Ages and the Dark Ages. The development of increased maritime prowess made longer and more frequent exploratory voyages possible, most notably the landfall in the Americas by Columbus in 1492. People's horizons were broadened, both literally and figuratively, and the flame of scientific inquiry was rekindled.

Lusk (1922) has pointed out that an understanding of the nature of air was essential to an adequate conception of nutrition. Two Renaissance thinkers, Leonardo da Vinci (1452–1519) and Santorio Sanctorius (1561–1636) made important observations relevant to this topic, which are fundamental to our current understanding of metabolism. Although the respiratory gases were not discovered until the late eighteenth century, some misty (nascent) insights were emerging. Da Vinci, a multitalented genius, noted at the end of the fifteenth century that no animal could live in an atmosphere that could not support a flame. Later, in 1614, Sanctorius, sometimes called the father of experiments in metabolism, published a celebrated account of his studies. Sitting day after day on his balance, he discovered that he lost weight during periods when he had taken in neither food nor drink, even though no urine or feces had passed from his body. He explained this loss as due to "insensible perspiration." (Actually, water had evaporated from his body.)

The Golden Age of Science

The seventeenth century marked the beginning of modern science and the use of the experimental method. Scientists invented important instruments during this period, enabling them to perform experiments that previously had been impossible. The eighteenth century marked the rise of modern chemistry. Important chemical discoveries were made that paved the way for discoveries relating to nutrition as well. Because of the nature of nutrition, the development of nutritional science is intimately interrelated with clinical medicine, the biological sciences, chemistry, and agriculture. It has been said that nutrition as a science began with Lavoisier, who integrated the previous findings on respiration and built upon earlier work to explain and quantify energy metabolism during the late 1800s. We owe our present understanding of nutrition to the experimental method, which scientists continue to use today, as they seek further knowledge.

BASIC CONCEPTS OF NUTRITION

Because of their dependence on food for survival, all people, by necessity, have had intimate contact and familiarity with it since the human race began. Yet, most of our knowledge of the nutritive value of food did not emerge until the twentieth century. Why did it take so long? The answer is that until the 1900s, the level of knowledge within those sciences which related to nutrition, and the necessary analytical tools, had not become sophisticated enough to identify and measure the different nutrients in foods. These advances were necessary in order to learn how nutrients were used in carrying on essential functions in the body. For this reason, the study of nutrition often is referred to as a twentieth-century science.

In studying food habits, it is important to understand at least the basic concepts of nutrition, so that one has a sound basis for evaluating them. By studying the food habits of people in the past and the ways in which their dietary patterns affected them, we can gain valuable insights regarding ideal eating practices for people today.

The basic concepts of nutrition were identified by the White House Conference on Food, Nutrition and Health in 1969 (White House Conference, Final Report 1970:151). Since then, they have served as guidelines for nutrition education programs in the United States. They are summarized (and simplified) as follows:

1. Nutrition is the way the body uses food. We eat to live, to grow, to keep healthy and well, and to get energy for work and play.

2. Food is made up of different nutrients needed for growth and health. Nutrients include proteins, carbohydrates, fats, minerals, and vitamins. All nutrients needed by the body are available through food. Many kinds and combinations of food can lead to a well-balanced diet. No single food has all the nutrients needed for good growth and health. Each nutrient has specific uses in the body. Most nutrients do their best work in the body when teamed with other nutrients.

3. All persons, throughout life, have need for the same nutrients, but in varying amounts. The amounts of nutrients needed are influenced by age, sex, body size, activity, state of health, and heredity.

4. The way food is handled influences the amount of nutrients in food, its safety, quality, appearance, taste, acceptability, and cost. Handling means anything that

happens to food while it is being grown, processed, stored, and prepared for eating. (Lowenberg et al. 1979:143)

How Does the Body Use Food?

Good nutrition depends not only on the ingestion of nutritious, wisely selected foods, but on their proper utilization in the body. Proper utilization, in turn, depends on optimum digestion, absorption, and metabolism.

Food contains six classes of nutrients: proteins, fats, carbohydrates, minerals, vitamins, and water. Once it has been chewed and swallowed, food passes from the mouth through the esophagus to the stomach. Most of the nutrients in this food, however, cannot be absorbed and used by the body in their initial forms. Only glucose, alcohol, some inorganic salts, water, and certain fats (short chain triglycerides) from foods or beverages can be absorbed immediately through the walls of the stomach or intestines. Proteins, and most fats and carbohydrates, must be broken down before absorption can take place.

This breakdown occurs through the combined action of digestive enzymes, chemicals contained in various digestive secretions (such as gastric juice and bile), along with the physical effects of chewing and peristalsis. The fiber in plant foods contain complex carbohydrates (polysaccharides) that go through the gastrointestinal tract essentially unchanged.

Through these actions, proteins become broken down to amino acids; fats become broken down to smaller entities such as monoglycerides, fatty acids, and glycerol, and complex carbohydrate (e.g., starch) is broken down to glucose. These smaller fragments (or "metabolic building blocks") are able to pass through the pores of the mucosal wall, ultimately entering the blood stream. Once in the blood stream, these entities become involved in a complex array of reactions known collectively as "metabolism," whereby the body obtains energy, builds and maintains tissue, and carries on other important functions.

Calories/Energy. Of the six classes of nutrients, only protein, fats, and carbohydrates provide energy (including heat) when they combine with oxygen in the body. Vitamins, minerals, and water do not supply energy directly, but they play an indirect role in energy production in that they aid in the metabolism of proteins, fats and carbohydrates. Per gram of pure nutrient ingested, the following net amounts of kilocalories (energy) are released: carbohydrates, 4; fats, 9; and proteins, 4 kilocalories.

Energy is expressed in kilocaries (Kcalories) obtained per gram of food. A kilocalorie is that amount of energy necessary to raise one kilogram (1,000 grams) of water one degree Centigrade. It should be noted that most foods are not pure carbohydrate, fat, or protein; often, a food may contain a mixture of two or all three of these nutrients. However, when one burns a substance that is pure carbohydrate, fat, or protein in the Atwater calorimeter, one obtains 4, 9, and 4 Kcalories of energy per gram, respectively. A gram is a unit of weight used in chemistry and is part of the metric system. It is 1/454 of a pound or 1/28 of an ounce. It can be seen that fats give us more than twice the calories per unit weight than either carbohydrate or protein. No wonder a diet high in fat is "fattening"! It is important to remember this fact when planning calorie-controlled diets.

Carbohydrates. These nutrients all contain carbon (C), hydrogen (H), and oxygen (O). Using the sun's rays as a source of energy, plants synthesize carbohydrate from the carbon dioxide in the air and water from the soil. Thus, through plants, carbohydrate plays an essential role as the chief source of energy for the animal kingdom, including the world's people. Most of the globe's food staples are rich in carbohydrate (e.g., corn, manioc, rice, sugar, taro, wheat, and other cereal grains).

The only carbohydrates that are not directly of plant origin are lactose, or milk sugar (found only in the milk of mammals), and glycogen (found in the liver and muscles of animals).

Lipids. These nutrients, like carbohydrates, contain C, H, and O, but in different combinations. Lipids include fatty acids, fats and oils, phospholipids, and sterols. They are widespread in nature, occurring both in animals and plants.

Since they constitute a concentrated source of energy, they serve as a reserve source of energy for animals and plants (especially in seeds), as well as a concentrated source of calories in the diet. Most of the fatty acids in human metabolism can be synthesized by the body. However, the exception is linoleic acid, a polyunsaturated fatty acid, which must be supplied by the diet. Hence, it is designated as an "essential" fatty acid.

Important global food sources of fat include meat, milk, poultry and eggs, nuts, and seed oils (e.g., corn, cottonseed, olive, sunflower, safflower, soybean, and others).

Proteins. These substances are unique in that, in addition to C, H, and O, they all contain nitrogen (N) also. Early chemists recognized that a common entity existed in all living things that was essential for life. For this reason, Gerardus Mulder proposed the name "protein" for this nitrogen-containing substance, derived from the Greek word "proteus," meaning "to come first."

Proteins are large molecules composed of building blocks called amino acids. Foods contain over 20 different amino acids, all of which are needed by the human organism. Some of these acids can be synthesized by the body from other nitrogen-containing molecules. However, 8 amino acids are referred to as essential because they can not be synthesized by the human body and must be supplied, preformed, by the diet. They are: isoleucine, leucine, lysine, methionine, phenylalanine, threonine, tryptophan, and valine. Those proteins which contain all of the essential amino acids are able to maintain life and support growth and are classified as complete.

Proteins lacking in one or more of these amino acids are designated as incomplete. In general, proteins from animal sources are complete (e.g., meat, fish, poultry, milk, and eggs). However, most proteins from vegetable (plant) sources are incomplete because they are lacking in one or more of four indispensable amino acids: lysine, methionine, threonine, and methionine. However, an adequate intake of essential amino acids still can be obtained by using complementary sources of vegetable protein, whose collective amino acid contents will compensate for individual deficiencies. For example, soybeans and corn are a good combination. Soybeans are good sources of lysine, threonine, and tryptophan but are relatively low in methionine, while corn, on the other hand, shows essentially an opposite amino acid pattern (Williams 1989:Appendix B).

Minerals. These inorganic substances, which must be provided by the diet, constitute about 4 percent of the body's weight. They serve two general functions: as structural constituents and as regulatory substances in various body processes. At present, seventeen mineral elements are known to be essential for human life, good health, and growth. Certain minerals, especially those which serve as constituents of hard and soft tissues (e.g., bones and teeth; muscle and nervous tissue) are present in appreciable amounts and comprise 0.05 percent or more of the body's weight. They are known as macrominerals. Those minerals which are needed in amounts of less than 0.05 percent are referred to as micronutrients, or trace elements. Of the macronutrients, calcium and phosphorus are present in the highest amounts (roughly 2 percent and 1 percent, respectively), followed by potassium, sulfur, sodium, chlorine, and magnesium. The microminerals include iron, manganese, copper, iodine, cobalt, zinc, chromium, selenium, molybdenum, and fluorine. Minute amounts of other minerals are also found in the body. They include silicon, vanadium, and nickel. But it is not yet certain whether their presence is purely happenstance or whether any of them actually perform specific biological functions in the body.

Vitamins. These organic compounds are necessary in small amounts for growth and maintenance of life and cannot be synthesized by the body. Thus, they must be supplied by the diet. Vitamins are classified as fat soluble or water soluble. The fat-soluble vitamins, A, D, E, and K, tend to be stored in the body, especially the liver, whereas water-soluble vitamins are stored to a much lesser extent. These latter vitamins include the members of the B-complex family and vitamin C. Vitamins are obtained through the consumption of a varied, balanced diet (see table 1.1).

Water. This nutrient is the most prevalent compound in the body, comprising about 65 percent of its weight. It is second only to oxygen in its importance to the body. All of the body processes, including its metabolic reactions, must take place in the presence of water. Without water, an individual may die within a few days. Once taken for granted, and omitted in nutrient classification schemes, water now is accorded its rightful status

Table 1.1
Food Guides

Food Guide	Food Groups	Daily Servings
Basic Four[1]	Milk	2
	Meat	2
	Vegetable, fruit	4
	Bread, cereal	4
Six Food Group Plan[2]	Breads, cereals, and other grain products	6–11
	Fruits	2–4
	Vegetables	3–5
	Meat, poultry, fish, and alternates	2–3
	Milk, cheese, and yogurt	2
	Fats, concentrated sweets, and alcoholic beverages[3]	Use sparingly

[1]USDA/ARS 1958.

[2]USDA/HNIS 1989.

[3]Foods in this category are called "Extras" because they are not necessary in the diet. They should be eaten only once in a while, within individual calorie limits.

as an essential nutrient. The sources of water are the fluids of the diet (preferably 1 to 1 1/2 quarts daily), the solid foods of the diet, and that water which is produced by the metabolism of the energy nutrients within the body's tissues.

Functions of Food

Food satisfies physiological, and also social and psychological needs (chapter 7). Physiologically, it has three functions: to furnish body fuel for energy, to provide material to build and maintain tissue, and to supply substances to regulate body processes. These needs are fulfilled by the nutrients found in food. Some foods are especially nutritious because they perform all three of these physiological roles. Others may contribute mainly to energy production.

Food Plans

How can one know whether one is choosing the correct foods for an adequate intake of energy and essential nutrients? For most of us, it simply is not practical to be consulting food composition tables when planning meals at home or when ordering from a menu at a restaurant! Aware of this problem, nutritionists over the years have developed practical, easily memorized food guides that enable even the busiest person to make wise food choices quickly, without the constant necessity of consulting tables.

In 1958, the Basic Four Food Group Plan was developed by nutritionists in the United States Department of Agriculture (USDA, ARS 1958). Over the next several decades, the Basic Four (with modifications) served as the most widely used food guide in the United States (Tables 1.1. and 6.1). This plan gives the minimum number of servings recommended daily for foods from each of the Four Food Groups (familiar to most Americans): milk, meat, fruits and vegetables, and breads and cereals. In 1989, in response to the need for a food guide that better reflected newer knowledge regarding the association of dietary excesses (e.g., fat, calories, sugar) with chronic degenerative diseases, the USDA developed a new, six-food group plan, with recommended ranges of servings (USDA, HNIS 1989) (table 1.1). The actual number of servings for each group is determined by an individual's age, level of activity, and other factors. In 1992, the USDA introduced this six-food group plan as a graphic, known as the Food Guide Pyramid (Food Technology 1992; USDA, HNIS 1992). Jointly adopted by the USDA and the United States Department of Health and Human Services (USDHHS), this graphic serves as a useful nutrition education tool. Like its predecessors, this plan is designed for individuals who are able to consume a general diet. The plan must be modified for people on special diets.

EVOLUTION AND HUMAN DIETARY NEEDS

The study of human evolution provides an important perspective on the ways in which the human body has developed and adapted over time. Along with changes in nutrition, there have been alterations in the body's metabolism and morphology (form and structure) in response to dietary modifications. Many of these changes have nutritional significance for people living today.

Types of Adaptations

Beneficial adaptations are geared toward survival. Those changes which enhance reproductive potential of the individual ultimately enhance the potential for survival of the group (Johnston 1982:56). Because of its adaptability, the human species has demonstrated an outstanding capacity to survive. In fact, Jane Underwood (1979:160) has noted that the human species occupies a broader range of environments than any other primate species. Man has been able to adapt to these diverse environments through positive behavioral, physiological, and genetic responses (Bryant, Courtney, Markesbery, and DeWalt, 1985:6–7).

While humans may react to an environmental challenge with all three types of changes, the rates at which they occur are quite different. The most immediate response will be behavioral, since that is the most rapid way of adapting to an environmental pressure. If behavioral responses alone are insufficient, they may be followed by physiological changes. If the environmental challenge continues over a long period, genetic adaptations might occur that would reinforce or even replace the original behavioral and physiological responses. Genetic adaptations are brought about by mutation. Genetically transmitted traits that confer a survival advantage and greater reproductive success will tend to increase within the population because individuals with these traits will be hardier and produce more offspring than those individuals lacking these traits.

The following scenario illustrates a situation in which all three mechanisms (behavioral, physiological, and genetic) might be involved. Suppose that the climate in the southern part of the United States suddenly became much warmer. The first response(s) would probably be to wear less clothing, to seek the shade, or to use more fans or air-conditioning. These adaptations are behavioral. If these responses proved insufficient, the normal level of perspiration probably would increase. This physiological response would enable most persons to cope successfully with the increased temperature. However, profuse sweating over an extended period could lead to a dangerous loss of water and salt. Therefore, if the hot climate persisted, those individuals with specific genetically transmitted traits which enabled them to adapt better than others to these conditions would be more likely to survive and reproduce. For example, individuals whose renal functions provided a more sensitive calibration of antidiuretic hormone (ADH) might lose less water through urination and thus enjoy a selective advantage. The increased renal retention of sodium could also confer a selective advantage. Individuals with a predisposition toward less body fat or a lower body metabolism would also be at an advantage in this warm environment.

Sometimes there can be an interaction of behavioral, physiological, and genetic responses at the same time. According to Carol Bryant et al. (1985: 13), such adaptations are complex and often difficult to sort out.

It must be emphasized that the very traits which enable populations to become better adapted to one environment may actually serve as a disadvantage under other conditions. For example, some nutritionists believe that the high prevalence of hypertension among African Americans today is a result of a (historic) genetic adaptation favoring increased salt (sodium) retention. In African habitats, high temperatures were common, and salt loss through perspiration was high. In the tropics, with diets relatively high in plant materials (and hence, relatively low in sodium), individuals with a genetic tendency toward higher sodium retention would enjoy a selective advantage. However, that same trait could be disadvantageous to African Americans today. Coupled with their typically high sodium intake, this adaptation could result in an unusually high degree of salt retention. The latter can be an important risk factor for the development of hypertension.

Evolving Nutritional Needs and Changing Food Sources

All forms of life have strikingly similar nutritional needs. However, these needs often are satisfied in different ways. Those nutrients which cannot be manufactured by the organism itself must be obtained from the environment (i.e., from the air, water, and food). Those nutritional needs which are fulfilled by oral ingestion (i.e., by food and water) are called dietary needs. Our present dietary needs are the product of a long history of evolutionary change.

Beginning dietary needs. The earliest forms of life are thought to have been one-celled bacteriumlike organisms that were capable of an autotrophic existence. In other words, they were able to manufacture all of the compounds needed for life from mineral salts, carbon dioxide, simple sources of nitrogen (ammonia, nitrates or nitrite) and water. However, over time, rare and random mutations occurred, producing organisms that lacked one or more of these synthetic capabilities. If the needed nutrient(s) were available from the environment, the organism would still be able to live and pass the trait on to succeeding generations. In fact, such mutations may even have conferred a selective advantage, since it reduced the total number of biochemical reactions necessary in cells, which already probably were overloaded with biosynthetic demands (Scrimshaw and Young 1980: 52). As a result, organisms evolved that were increasingly dependent on external sources of nutrients for existence.

The first one-celled animals, who appeared about 1 billion years ago, lacked a number of the biosynthetic capabilities found in plant cells, in particular the power of photosynthesis. Through this latter process, plants convert the energy of sunlight into energy-rich compounds that serve as the powerhouse for the cell's activities. Over millennia, through mutations, animals evolved that were even more dependent on external sources of energy and nutrients for their existence.

The human as animal. Humans share various traits with other members of the animal kingdom who evolved from these common ancestors. (The taxonomic classification of humans is shown in Table 1.2.) One of these characteristics is that they share certain common nutritional needs. In addition to minerals, all animals need an exogenous source of certain carbon compounds to sustain life. These include amino acids, carbohydrates (for energy), certain fatty acids, and vitamins, although the degree of dependence will vary from species to species. All animals also must have water. In most animals, water is obtained from an external source, rather than through internal synthesis. Ruminants, however, do not require dietary sources of certain vitamins and amino acids because their intestinal flora are able to digest cellulose, from which they synthesize various vitamins and amino acids, which then becomes available to the animal.

Another example of differing dependence on vitamins involves vitamin

Table 1.2
Taxonomic Classification of Humans

Kingdom—Animal

Phylum—Chordata

Class—Mammalia

Order—Primate (anthropoids, prosimians)

Suborder—Anthropoidea (humans, apes, monkeys)

Superfamily—Hominoidea (humans, apes)

Family—Hominidae (humans)

Genus—Homo

Species—sapiens

C. Humans and most other primates and the guinea pig are the only mammals that require a dietary source of vitamin C. Other species are able to synthesize this vitamin from glucose. It has been hypothesized that a mutation occurred millions of years ago in certain mammals, altering the enzyme responsible for converting L-gulonic acid to L-ascorbic acid, the terminal reaction in a series of steps whereby L-ascorbic acid is produced from glucose. Fortunately, this mutation was not lethal, because the affected species were able to obtain generous quantities of this nutrient from various plant sources in the environment. Nevin Scrimshaw and Vernon Young (1980:52) have noted Linus Pauling's suggestion that this mutation indeed may have been advantageous, since it freed glucose to be used by the body for energy.

The human as omnivorous mammal. All mammals have basically the same nutritional needs. However, not all mammals require a dietary source of specific nutrients. Humans, like most mammals (Table 1.2), are omnivores, that is, they take food from more than one trophic level (Milton 1987:93). In other words, they eat foods of both vegetable and animal origin. Different species satisfy their specific dietary requirements in diverse ways, choosing from a wide range of foods. Moreover, the digestive capabilities of omnivorous mammals show differences as well. In general, there is a discernible positive correlation between the specialized diet and gut morphology within a given species.

The human as primate. Humans are members of the highest order of mammals, the primates (Table 1.2). Like other members of this group, they developed special traits that set them apart from other animals because of their adaptation to a tree-dwelling existence. (For an extensive discussion of these traits, see Bryant et al. 1985:17–18).

The omnivorous diet of ancestral hominids undoubtedly was similar in some respects to that of other primates, particularly the diet of other hominoids (i.e., the great apes: gorillas, orangutans, and chimpanzees) (Milton 1987:94).

By the time the primate line evolved, presumably by the Middle Paleocene period, a wide variety of dietary opportunities had already become available, because of the adaptive radiation and eventual dominance of angiosperms (flowering plants with seeds enclosed in an ovary), which had occurred during the preceding Cretaceous epoch (Regal 1977). Available foods included the insects that pollinated angiosperm flowers, in addition to the pollen, nectar, fruits and foliage of the angiosperms themselves (Eisenberg 1981).

The available data, including observations of present-day primates, would indicate that primates are omnivores of a particular type. That is, they focus primarily on plant foods, augmented by only small amounts of animal matter. Strong support for this view is provided by the gut morphology of the primate. The normative primate gut is relatively unspecialized, indicative that primates, particularly the anthropoids (including humans), traditionally have focused on very high-quality plant foods that are not extensively fibrous or lignified, supplementing them with second trophic level foods (Milton 1987: 97–98).

The hominoid as anthropoid. All members of the Hominoidea (anthropoids) (Table 1.2) show the same basic gut pattern. According to Milton (1987:100), hominoids have a simple acid stomach, a small cecum terminating in a true appendix, and a well-sacculated colon.

Despite these similarities in gut morphology among the hominoids, there are notable differences between humans and other hominoids when relative gut proportions are compared. In humans, by far the greatest gut volume is found in the small intestine (≥ 56 percent), with relatively lower volume (≥ 23 percent) in the colon. Pongids, on the other hand, show essentially opposite trends. Also, the size of the human gut relative to body mass is small in comparison with most other anthropoids (Milton 1987: 100–101). According to this author, the strong development of both the cecum and colon (as in pongids) are generally good predictors of diets high in plant fiber (99–101). Pongids (e.g., gorillas and orangutans) consume large quantities of leaves and other plant parts not regularly eaten by humans.

There can be little doubt that the ancestral line giving rise to the Hominoidea superfamily and ultimately to hominids (humans) was markedly herbivorous (104). Results of analyses of rehydrated human coprolites have indicated a consumption of up to 130 grams of plant fiber per day until relatively recently (Kliks 1978). In addition, human coprolites contain undigested residues of animal tissue, including such materials as bones, teeth, hair, feathers, keratinized skin, fish scales, and insect cuticle. At times, these animal substances contribute more than 10 percent of the total weight of undigested residues. The ingestion of these food components indicate a minimum of food preparation involved at this level of development. Also, it suggests that eating was a fiercely competitive activity, where food had to be consumed quickly, lest it be snatched away by a peer.

Katharine Milton (1987:101) cites a variety of animal studies which indicate that increases in energy requirements without a decrease in dietary quality will increase the size of the small intestine and decrease the colon. She notes that present-day proportions of the human gut in technological societies indicate utilization of nutritionally dense, energetically concentrated foods.

It would appear that the relatively small size of the human colon represents a derived trait, rather than the ancestral condition of Hominoideae. William Hill (1949) has pointed out that the colon of the human neonate is more similar to that of pongids than is the case for mature individuals. Humans show regression of the colon as they mature, whereas pongids show elongation, particularly of the left colon.

The human as hominid. The first hominids (the Australopithecines) emerged between 4 and 3.75 million years ago (Philbeam 1984:94). These early humans are believed to have evolved in a grassland setting, from primates who had migrated there when tropical forests began to dry up because of global climatic change. In this environment, both plant and animal foods of high quality would be more patchily distributed, over both space and time, than in tropical forests (Milton 1981). Thus, early hominids would have been forced to forage over broad areas, if they were concentrating on higher-quality, more digestible foods. Such circumstances would require a degree of mobility much more likely to be attained by walking on two legs rather than all fours. In fact, Peter Rodman and Henry McHenry (1980) have hypothesized that selective pressures related to travel efficiency between widely dispersed food sources in a savannah setting may have stimulated the adaptation of bipedalism in the hominid line. In addition to increasing mobility, bipedalism freed the hands for food-getting activities. These hominids had not yet discovered stone tools, judging from their absence in association with australopithecine remains (Philbeam 1984: 95).

From homo erectus to modern human. A more advanced hominid appeared about 1.5 millions years ago: Homo erectus. The first widely distributed hominid, its remains have been found in three continents—Africa, Asia, and Europe. Homo erectus was relatively big brained and used crude, all-purpose implements, including stone hand axes (Harris 1980:73).

Homo erectus gradually evolved into Homo sapiens. An early form of this species emerged about 250,000 years ago, while modern Homo sapiens appeared about 35,000 years ago. Homo sapiens showed changes which have continued until the present: increased brain size, enhanced intellectual capabilities, more sophisticated tools, and more complex forms of organization (Bryant et al. 1985:29). Under the Ice Age conditions that existed during the period of early Homo sapiens, hunting continued to play an important role (Johnston 1982:300). Associated with the evolution of modern Homo sapiens was the development of new and more sophisticated tools and weapons, including the bow and arrow, spear thrower, needles with eyes, axes, spoons, stone saws, antler hammers, shovels, and pestles (Bryant et al. 1985:29).

FOR FURTHER READING

Bryant, C.A., A. Courtney, B.A. Markesbery, and K.M. DeWalt. 1985. *The cultural feast.* St. Paul, MN: West Publishing Company.

Johnston, F.E. 1982. *Physical anthropology.* Dubuque, IA: Wm. C. Brown Company.

Lowenberg, M.E., E.N. Todhunter, E.D. Wilson, J.R. Savage, and J.L. Lubawski. 1979. *Food and people* (3rd ed.). New York: John Wiley and Sons.

Milton, K. 1987. Primate guts and gut morphology: implications for hominid evolution. In M. Harris and E. Ross (eds.), *Food and evolution* (93–115). Philadelphia: Temple University Press.

Scrimshaw, N., and V. Young. 1980. The requirements of human nutrition. In A.L. Tobias and P.J. Thompson (eds.), *Issues in nutrition for the 1980s* (50–61). Monterey, CA: Wadsworth Health Sciences Division.

United States Department of Agriculture, Human Nutrition Information Service. 1989. *Preparing foods and planning menus using the dietary guidelines.* Home and Garden Bulletin 232–8:11. Washington, DC: USGPO.

———. 1992. *The food guide pyramid.* Home and Garden Bulletin 252. Washington, DC: USGPO.

Williams, S.R. 1989. *Nutrition and diet therapy* (6th ed.). St. Louis: Times Mirror/ Mosby College Publishing.

2

The Search for Food

Securing sufficient food to satisfy the needs of its members is essential to the existence of any society. Throughout the human experience, people have had to devote a great deal of time and effort to obtaining an adequate food supply. Humans also have endeavored continuously to increase the reliability of their subsistence, thereby increasing the overall security of their existence (Hayden 1981a).

METHODS OF SECURING FOOD

Methods for obtaining food fall into two major categories, food gathering and food production. Food gathering involves the utilization of the resources of the environment, just as they exist, without any attempts to improve or increase the available supply. In contrast, food production involves attempts to alter and improve the existing food supply through such techniques as the planting of seeds and care of plants (gardening) or the domestication and care of animals (animal husbandry). The latter approach usually results in a greater food supply from a given area than by employing food gathering alone. It is widely accepted that the first people were food gatherers, and that this stage has persisted throughout human history. Food production, on the other hand, evolved late in the human experience.

The two categories of food procurement are not mutually exclusive. As humans began to produce food, they did not abandon gathering activities,

Figure 2.1
Cereal Grains Are the Primary Food in the World

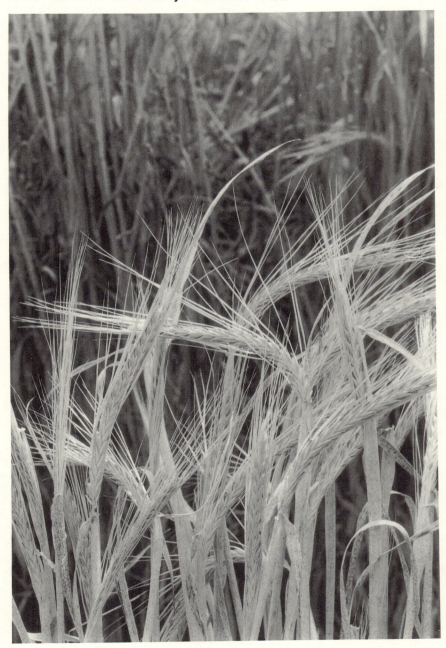

Agricultural Research Service, USDA

but continued to use them for augmenting their food supply. In fact, even advanced technological societies today still engage in food gathering, in addition to food production. Foods such as wild rice, cranberries from bogs, wild berries, brazil nuts, fish, and other foods continue to be harvested, and such activities are referred to collectively as extractive industries.

Food Gathering

The term "food gathering" as used here refers to all kinds of food-getting activities in which there is no attempt to increase the amount of food available. The term "food foraging" is used to describe rudimentary food gathering where plant and/or animal material is assembled using little or no special technology (Beals and Hoijer 1971). These activities can be either aimless and random or goal oriented. Hunting, fishing, and collecting, on the other hand, denote a more technical level of food gathering. In these three latter endeavors, there is a purposive search for game, fish, or food plants, respectively, employing special (albeit frequently simple) implements.

Food foraging. Food gathering undoubtedly began with simple foraging, which still continues today, even in modern societies. For example, picking blueberries in the woods, by hand, would be considered foraging. To begin with, it is thought that early hominids consumed an unprocessed, primarily vegetarian diet. This fare was supplemented with smaller amounts of animal foods (such as insects and larva) that were often ingested almost coincidentally (e.g., in a ripe piece of fruit). Thus, the human has always been, at least to some degree, an omnivore. During the Late Miocene to early Pleistocene period, there was a shift from this diet to one that relied on nonoral food preparation techniques and significant proportions of meat (Gordon 1987:3; Milton 1987).

As a food forager, essentially without tools, man at the hominid stage likely obtained meat by scavenging and engaging in various opportunistic activities. Slow-moving, small animals could easily be killed, even with the hands, then eaten. Larger animals would have been beyond his capabilities, unless the animal were sick, wounded, or already dead. Therefore, it is thought that scavenging and eating carrion (dead animals) probably represented important sources of meat for the early food forager. Some anthropologists believe that scavenging may have been a transitional phase between foraging and hunting (Gordon 1987:9).

Early foragers lacked containers, so they tended to eat their food where they found it, rather than transporting it back to camp. Thus, they tended to be nomadic and "on the move." This pattern continued until emergent human forms (e.g., Australopithecines) developed technology (Beals and Hoijer 1971:195–96). Their numbers were limited by the amount of food available in the season of greater scarcity, since they lacked the means to preserve or store food. Humans have been food foragers throughout most of their history; for example, for the several hundred thousand years of the Paleolithic period.

More specialized techniques. Early food foraging activities later were expanded to include the more specialized techniques of hunting, fishing, and collecting. These latter activities involved the deliberate search for, and procurement, of game, fish, and plant foods, using special tools or implements. Kathleen Gordon (1987:3) has suggested that specialized hunting and gathering strategies may have begun with Homo erectus and subsequently improved. Both continue to be used today.

Historically, no food-gathering culture has tended to rely solely on any one of the three methods of food gathering. But, usually, one method will take precedence over the others in providing the major portion of the diet. The dominant technique usually is determined by the character of the environment (including the staple food of a given locale).

Collecting. The garnering of wild vegetable products with the aid of specialized techniques is termed collecting. Because of the poor preservability of such foods, along with the relatively quick deterioration of the types of tools and baskets customarily used for these activities, collecting assemblages have been underrepresented in the various assemblages that have been discovered in caves and other archeological finds. Therefore, the actual role of collecting in early subsistence undoubtedly has been greatly underrated. Because of the tenuous nature of these artifacts, it probably will never be possible to determine exactly when humans advanced from pure foraging to collecting plant foods. In fact, it is highly probable that man always has employed rudimentary tools of some sort; primates today have been observed using small twigs as implements for the removal of insect and larval material from plant foods.

In addition to their use of complex and specialized technologies, collectors tend to differ from (plant) foragers in three important ways (Beals and Hoijer 1971:222–23):

1. They have techniques to process many plants inedible in their raw state to make them palatable and nourishing.
2. Their efficient collecting techniques permit accumulating a reserve of storable plant foods.
3. They have adequate containers for transport and storage.

The evolutionary significance of the advent of containers and storage technology has been emphasized by Norge Jerome (1981:38), Waldo Wedel (1964), and David Yesner (1987:295). Jerome has pointed out the importance of the development of two related innovations in the New World, particularly among the Woodland Indians in what is now the United States. These included the development of the storage pit and the development of pottery (Wedel 1964:205). The storage pit, usually a bell-shaped hole dug in the ground and lined with grass, was used to store grains and nuts that were gathered. With pottery, water could be stored, and meats and grain could be cooked by methods other than roasting.

Today, there are no people so primitive as to be dependent upon wild vegetable foods alone. All nonhorticultural people possess adequate tools and weapons for both hunting and fishing, as well. Nevertheless, studies of modern hunting and gathering peoples have shown an unexpectedly high reliance on vegetable foods. Although hunting is more dramatic than collecting, and meat is highly prized, it nevertheless represents an unpredictable subsistence strategy. For most hunter-gatherers living today, it constitutes a relatively small proportion of the diet. For example, studies of the !Kung San people of Botswana (Lee 1968; 1979) showed that vegetable foods contributed approximately 67 percent to the total diet (by calories), with meat from hunting by the males being brought home only about one day in four. Other studies of modern hunter-gatherers have shown much the same pattern, where the most common and reliable subsistence strategy is based on a high consumption of vegetable foods (Hayden 1981b; Meggitt 1962; Woodburne 1968), collected primarily by women and children. Even for modern hunters, hunting is an unpredictable food source (Gordon 1987:12).

Historically, plant foods have been collected primarily, but not exclusively, by women, often with their children (Dahlberg 1981:1–33). Children have been uniquely helpful in collecting activities. Smaller and more agile than adult women, they could climb trees with greater ease and could shake down nuts and fruits for the women to gather. Also, because of their smaller size, they were closer to the ground. Hence, they could pick up fallen bounty more easily.

Most modern collectors use fruits, grains, seeds, roots, and tubers; relatively little use is made of shoots, stalks, or leaves, which form a major part of the diet of the gorilla. They tend to specialize in one staple. For example, California Indians depend primarily on the acorn, while their neighbors in the Great Basin (between the Rockies and the Sierras) use a variety of small seeds in spring and summer and piñon nuts in fall and winter. Piñon nuts are seeds from the cones of the piñon pine, collected during a short period, usually late autumn. Seri Indians of Sonora, Mexico, harvest the grain of a grass that grows in the Gulf of California, between continental Mexico and Baja, California. It is the only known instance of grain from the sea used as a human food source.

Not all environments are equally rewarding to collectors. Most of the people classed as collectors today are found in the Americas. But, surprisingly, they are not found in tropical America, although the American tropics are richer in edible plants than those of other regions. Instead, the majority of them live in the semiarid regions of North America, extending from eastern Washington and Oregon to central Mexico, and from the coast of California to the Gulf of Mexico. Plants here tend to produce seeds high in starch, with a hard outer shell or coating. Collecting as a livelihood first developed in what some archaeologists call the desert cultures of western North America, appearing at least by 8000 B.C., following rather shortly the early hunting cultures of these areas (Beals and Hoijer 1971: 223–25).

Collecting is not a simple technology. It requires great knowledge of the environment and plant characteristics, as well as special implements and methods for preparing wild foods. The seed beater, essentially a threshing implement, is an important tool. Mortars and pestles also have been indispensable for collectors and horticulturists, for grinding seeds into a flour or meal.

Hunting. The hunting and gathering societies peaked during the last great Ice Age (the 4th Glacier Period and Interglacial Period), about 18,000 years ago. Hunting involves the pursuit of animals using special tools and traditionally has been carried out by men. However, women also engage in this activity (Estioko-Griffin and Griffin 1981:121–51). Hunting societies, by definition, depend upon game for the bulk of their food supply. But, within this category, great differences may exist.

The Plains Indians traditionally have focused on bison, when available, otherwise going to smaller animals. As bison hunters they were forced to kill large numbers at certain times of the year and then preserve the meat or to follow the bison herds in their seasonal migrations. The Eskimos depend primarily upon sea mammals such as the seal and walrus in wintertime but move inland in summer to hunt the caribou and collect cloudberries.

Among the most important missile weapons employed in hunting are the spear, harpoon, and bow and arrow. Used less frequently are the sling, bola, boomerang, and spear-thrower. In modern societies, the most widely known missile weapon is the gun, first used by the Arabs in North Africa in the 1300s.

The use of missile weapons is possible only if the hunter gets within effective range of his quarry. Early peoples developed great skill in stalking animals or in lying in wait for them at watering places and along game trails (Figure 2.2). They also learned to imitate mating calls as a means of attracting animals.

Group activities often are more effective than individual effort. For example, among the Nisenans of California, several hunters may station themselves beside game trails while others drive deer in their direction. Or, they set fire to the grass in a great circle and either kill the game as it escapes through the flames or recover the game killed by the fire. Small game also

Figure 2.2
Paleo-Indian Hunter Stalks His Prey

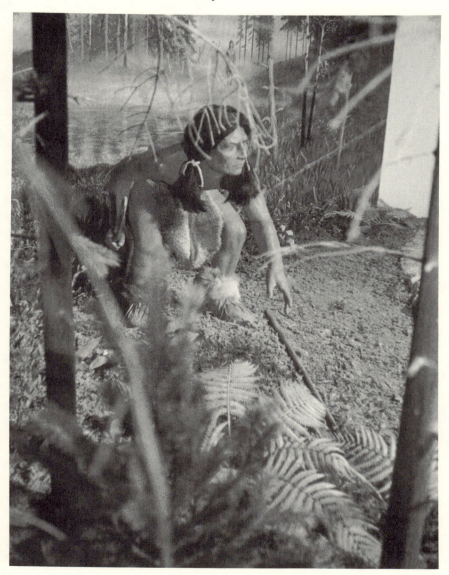

Press Gazette Collection of the Neville Public Museum of Brown County

may be hunted as a group activity, employing some of these techniques. Rabbit hunts still are common in the midwestern United States during winter.

Pitfalls, nets, snares, and traps are used everywhere. The Yaquis of northwest Mexico catch deer with rope snares attached to bent saplings that jerk the animal's forefeet into the air and hold it until the hunter arrives. Small animals and birds are often caught with nets and snares. Although most hunting people have dogs, not all employ them in hunting.

Many hunters preserve meat either by drying, salting, or both. Preservation is especially important where game affords the main food supply yet is only seasonally in abundance. The Plains Indians dry and smoke meat. In addition, they often make a highly concentrated and nourishing food called pemmican (dried meat pounded to a power and mixed with fat), which has excellent keeping qualities.

Other people, particularly in warm climates, do not preserve meat, but eat it as soon as possible (e.g., the Yaquis of Sonora, Mexico). The ability of some hunting people to gorge themselves on meat has been noted in many places, especially among the Eskimos. Where transportation is simple or lacking, conservation of any amount of meat often is impractical, and it must be eaten with dispatch. In such situations, it is customary to share the kill with the immediate group or with neighboring villages. Historically, the ability to provide a feast, with animals obtained by hunting, has brought man much prestige. And eating in a group also has given people much pleasure; in general, we prefer not to eat alone.

Fishing. According to Frances Dahlberg (1981:15), it is unclear what role, if any, fish played in the evolutionary past. Since fish bones and gathered foods do not preserve well, fishing and gathering (collecting) are more difficult to document in the past than hunting. This fact also may explain, in part, why fishing techniques do not appear to be as old as those for hunting (Beals and Hoijer 1971:219). Anthropologists agree that significant use of fish does not seem to have occurred until relatively late in the prehistoric record, both in the Old and New worlds (Osborn 1977; Yesner 1987:285). According to Gordon (1987:22), "Marine foods, including shellfish, fish, and marine mammals rarely figure very significantly in Middle and early Upper Pleistocene site remains." There seems to be no evidence of groups dependent primarily on fishing until postglacial times (Beals and Hoijer 1987:237). One factor may have been that during the large game era (chapter 4), an emphasis on fishing would have been incompatible with the nomadic lifestyle of the hunter.

Obviously, in order for a society to utilize fish as a primary source of subsistence, it had to be locally plentiful. Therefore, availability must always have been a precondition in determining the use of fish. Further, the degree of fish use seems to have been positively influenced directly by the degree of scarcity of other foods, such as game and plants.

The late use of marine resources also could be explained on the basis of optimal foraging theory (Yesner 1987:286–91). (This theory suggests that the likelihood of a resource being exploited is related to the nutrient density of that resource compared with the energy required to obtain it.) During most of the Pleistocene period, fish could have represented high-cost, low-benefit "secondary" resources. At that time, large game were plentiful and served as a primary dietary staple. But the progressive extinction and subsequent loss of these "valuable" megafauna during the Upper Paleolithic period is thought to have triggered the use of other previously underutilized resources, despite lower net yields. During the early Holocene, this meant that mainly smaller terrestrial resources became exploited. However, they became progressively scarce during mid-Holocene times, when climatic changes resulted in greater resource seasonality and increasingly patchy environments. Marine resources became very attractive under such circumstances. Not only were they nutrient-dense; they were most available in late winter and spring, at the very times when plant foods were least productive and animal foods were least accessible. Especially under such seasonal conditions, the development of storage technology in the late Pleistocene and early Holocene times obviously played an important role in the development of fishing in the Old World (295). The storability of seafoods—primarily through drying, smoking, salting, or freezing (where possible)—greatly enhances their reliability as a food resource.

The pattern of delayed adoption of marine resources is observable worldwide. When the adoption of fish food has occurred, it has resulted in a more sedentary lifestyle and increased population densities. Population growth, in turn, may force an even greater, often irreversible, commitment to a marine diet, similar to that which occurred with the adoption of agriculture (304).

It is apparent that, generally, fish as a food has been underused by man. The fact that fish are available does not always mean that they are used. This food behavior has been explained by lack of technology, other resources, and taboos. Various cultures forbid the eating of fish, including many Indians of the Plains and Southwest. Although many peoples use fish to supplement their diet, relatively few people build their subsistence around the use of it. Even coastal people who spend much of their time fishing often secure a considerable portion of their food by trade from inland dwellers in return for fish. Among the people most dependent on fish are those of the northern Pacific, especially in areas where salmon occur, or in the case of Eskimos, who hunt sea mammals (whale and seal).

The gathering of shellfish or mollusks (snails, oysters, and clams), which are soft invertebrates with a shell, afford an important source of food for many coastal peoples and involves very simple technology. Essentially, the only tool needed is a hardwood chisel, to pry the mollusks off the rocks. Often, this work is performed mainly by women and tends to be categorized as collecting. Fishing, on the other hand, usually involves a complex and varied technology and is most commonly carried on by men. The exception is small line fishing, often done by women and children, usually in small streams near the camp.

Spears and harpoons are used in many parts of the world. Nets, traps, and weirs are commonly used worldwide (Figure 2.3). Serious hook and line fishing seems to be confined mainly to the peoples of Oceania and the shores of the Pacific. Occasionally, the bow and arrow are used.

One of the most widespread methods of fishing is with the use of poisons or stupefacients, that is, substances which stun or paralyze the fish. In quiet pools or streams, or in tidal lagoons, this method can produce large quantities of fish with relatively little effort. However, it usually calls for the cooperation of several people. This technique is used widely throughout the tropics and is nearly as common in the temperate zones of North America and Asia. The poisons used are usually harmless to humans and come from a wide variety of plants suggesting intensive, thorough, and long-term experimentation with the environment.

Characteristics of Food-gathering Societies

Although food-gathering cultures vary, they tend to have certain common characteristics, summarized as follows.

1. Population density is usually low. Exceptions to this rule occur only in societies like those of the North Pacific coast or the Great Plains of America, where people live in areas especially favorable to collecting, hunting, or fishing. It is believed that as long as humans remained primarily hunter-gatherers, the world's total population never exceeded 5 to 10 million.

2. Food-gathering societies usually are small and isolated. They tend to move continuously or at frequent intervals from place to place to place in search of wild plants and animals. In other words, they usually are nomadic, in contrast to the more sedentary food producers.

3. Food gatherers are organized primarily into self-sufficient family groups, or more often, as loose confederations of families. Accordingly, their mechanisms of self-control and interaction are based more on kinship than on political organization.

4. Food gatherers today are found mainly in remote or marginal areas, where they presumably have been driven by the larger and more powerful food-producing societies. As a result, they tend to be slow to change, retaining certain patterns of culture that have long disappeared elsewhere.

5. Food gatherers have virtually no control over their food supply.

6. It is thought that the food gatherer of 1 1/2 million years ago practiced sharing, communal living, some division of labor, and tool making. (Leakey 1981:92–95)

Figure 2.3
Smelt Fishing, with Net

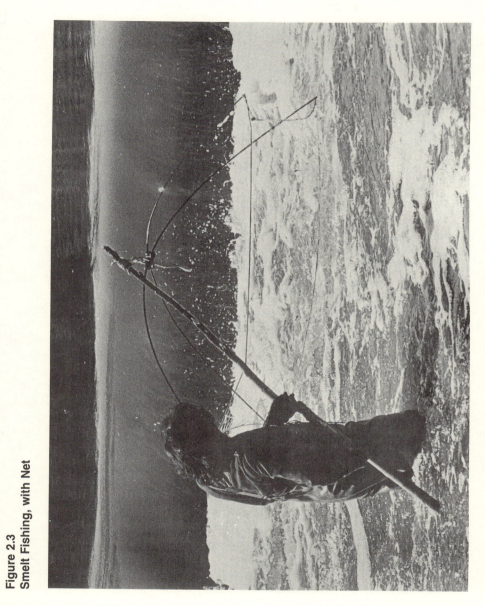

Food Production

It has been said that throughout history, great ideas have emerged in the minds of people in different parts of the world at the same time. This general observation certainly holds true for the development of food production, which began during the Upper Paleolithic period. This transition from dependence on the gathering of food as found in nature, to controlling the food supply by producing it, actually took place late in human history. And it evolved over thousands of years. It first began to occur in the more advanced societies throughout the world between 9 and 12 thousand years ago, when people began to domesticate plants and animals for food. In the Old World, the fossil record shows the beginnings of agriculture (horticulture) and animal husbandry by about 8000 B.C., with indications that an agrarian-based economy had become well established by 5000 B.C. (Braidwood and Howe 1960; Lamberg-Karlovsky and Sabloff 1979). Food producing spread into Europe from the Near East, while, in Africa and Asia, centers of domestication developed separately (Reed 1977). Three centers were involved in the independent development of food production in the New World: MesoAmerica, South America, and eastern North America (Smith 1989:1566–67).

Food production is viewed as a landmark development in the human experience that laid the foundations of modern civilization. However, Jack Harlan has noted that agriculture was not an invention or a discovery, nor was it as revolutionary as scholars believed in Nikolai Vavilov's day (during the first half of this century). In fact, "it was adopted slowly and with reluctance . . . (evolving) through an extension and intensification of what people had been doing for a long time" (1976:89).

With the development of food production, food gathering continued also, and still persists today. In fact, a few contemporary peoples still engage in food foraging, while virtually all societies continue to use the techniques of hunting, fishing, and collecting in varying degrees to obtain food. Food production probably evolved gradually as outgrowths of specialized food gathering strategies (e.g., hunting, fishing, and collecting).

The production of food involves those techniques by which the food supply ideally is increased, and controlled, at least to some extent. The leading food production technologies consist of horticulture, animal husbandry, and agriculture.

Horticulture. The shift in emphasis from food getting to food production most likely began with the domestication of plants by collectors, since they were so intimately involved with plant life. Moreover, the first horticulturists were probably women, given their traditionally close association with collecting (Beals and Hoijer 1971:239). Horticulture may have begun initially by accident, in several ways. Seeds could have dropped inadvertently onto the ground when women and children returned to camp with the day's "collected loot." Also, there is much evidence that early peoples discarded food refuse outside their caves and other dwellings. These "kitchen middens" undoubtedly contained seeds, which later sprouted and grew into plants, which then bore fruit. It is easy to envision that people soon began to recognize that having food-bearing plants right outside one's dwelling had definite advantages. It provided a more secure supply and saved both time and energy by reducing the number of collecting excursions necessary. As a result, humans probably soon began to place seeds deliberately in the ground close to their living quarters.

Horticulture has been described as "agriculture on a small scale." The term "horticulture" is usually applied to the cultivation of domestic plants for food and other purposes without the use of a plow. It implies the use of a digging stick, hoe, or hoelike tool made of wood, shell, or bone. Initially, a wooden digging stick was used, which might be something as simple as a large twig or limb of a tree. (Such rudimentary sticks still are used today in primitive "slash-and-burn" cultures.) Later, in addition to wood, shell and bone were used. Such tools would be suitable only for light cultivation. Many of these tools, especially those made of wood, did not survive. (For that reason, the archeological record of Middle to Upper Paleolithic plant utilization is very scanty compared with faunal debris [e.g., animal bones].)

Later, with the advent of metallurgy, these perishable tools became supplemented in certain societies by hoes and spades made of metal. These implements were capable of turning over the soil sufficiently for larger scale farming.

Animal husbandry. The raising of animals for food, or animal husbandry, has been associated both with pastoralism (herding of domestic animals) and nomadism. Early attempts at raising and caring for animals, of necessity, involved a nomadic lifestyle, because of the need to move from place to place to find adequate grazing opportunities for the flocks of sheep and goats. Gordon (1987:27) has suggested that in the Near East, animal husbandry began at about the same time as incipient agriculture. Robert Braidwood (1960) estimates these beginnings of food production at somewhere between 9,000 and 11,000 years ago. Gordon points out that "the earliest stages are difficult to detect, because the species eventually domesticated were present and heavily used before any morphological evidence of domestication appears" (1987:27). Abundant remains of sheep, goats, cattle, horses, and wolves associated with the Karim Shahir culture of the Zagros (Braidwood 1960; Braidwood and Howe 1960) indicate an early stage of animal domestication. The practice of animal husbandry, along with horticulture, encouraged mankind to become more sedentary.

The number of domesticated animals is far smaller than that of domesticated plants. The first domesticated animal was the dog. Based on a growing body of molecular data, along with the striking physiological and behavioral similarities between the two species, it now is almost certain that the ancestor of the domestic dog was the gray wolf (Morey 1994:339). This author notes that skeletal remains of early dogs from various archaeological sites, worldwide, would indicate that their domestication began in the late Pleistocene era, as early as 14,000 years ago. Thus, canid domestication must have taken place amongst people who still were hunter-gatherers, occurring independently, and in different regions (336;339). The general consensus among scholars is that the dog served mainly as a companion, protector, and hunting aid to early man, and only rarely as a food source.

What animal was the second to be domesticated? It appears that no single animal can claim this distinction. The finding of remains of several types of animals associated with the Karim Shahir culture (Braidwood and Howe 1960) indicates that a number of animals were becoming domesticated at about the same time.

What motivated animal domestication? Domestication of animals for meat seems likely, as well as for beasts of burden. Milking seems to be a later development than animal husbandry per se. Cave sites in Northern Iran indicate that goats were first raised for milk and meat; sheep raising followed, then the pig and ox (Coon 1951). The horse (a native of the Western Hemisphere) emigrated across the Bering Straits to the Eastern Hemisphere during the later Pleistocene (Crosby 1972:18), where it was used by early Asiatic nomads for transportation, milk, and blood. Many peoples, including some contemporary groups, eat their domestic animals only on rare ceremonial occasions. This practice suggests that, historically, the most prized role of meat may have been that of a religious offering (chapter 8).

Donkeys seem very likely to have been developed first in North Africa and cattle in southeast Asia. Sheep and goats come from the highlands of western Asia between Asia Minor and the Hindu Kush, where three wild forms occur. Reindeer are considered by many to be the last major animal to be domesticated. Chickens are native to Southeast Asia.

The beginning of animal domestication in America is not known. The turkey was present in Arizona and New Mexico by at least A.D. 700. The dog appears to have become domesticated much earlier, since skeletal remains of a dog were found in Idaho, dating to 11000 B.C. (Harlan 1976: 61).

The American Indians, in general, had many fewer domesticated animals than did Old World peoples. For one thing, the number of animals amenable to domestication was much smaller in the Western Hemisphere. The small number and inferior quality of domesticated animals in America were a severe handicap to the development of American Indian cultures. Although they used dogs to carry packs or pull a travois, Indians had limited transportation capabilities until the arrival of whites. Horses had existed in the Western Hemisphere since some unknown, early time but had died off sometime during the late Pleistocene (Crosby 1972:18). Thus, the Indians in the New World were without horses until they were re-introduced to the Western Hemisphere by Columbus in 1493 (80). Although horses have been used by man for meat, they have been kept primarily for riding (e.g., amongst pastoralists), general transportation, as a beast of burden, and for milk and blood. Like cows, they appear to have been commonly regarded as more valuable "on the hoof" than killed for meat.

Agriculture. The term "agriculture" is sometimes applied to all types of cultivation, including horticulture. More correctly, it should be used to define the raising of plants with the use of the plow (a mechanized spade) and draft animals, to augment human labor. Ralph Beals and Harry Hoijer have noted that true agriculture is of Old World origin and did not exist in the New World before European contact. The first types of plow were made of wood. But even these simple, early forms represented an important technological advance, since they enabled one person to cultivate a larger area and produce more foods than was possible by gardening. The plow served to prepare the soil, after which seeds (often wheat, barley, and rye) could be sown by broadcasting. The seeds then would be worked into the soil by dragging a brush (or later, a wooden drag harrow) through the seeded area (Beals and Hoijer 1971:276).

With the development of iron technology (chapter 3), plows and harrows began to be made of metal. This type of intensive agriculture was brought to the New World by the European colonists. Agriculture involving the use of the plow along with draft animals still is practiced in many parts of the world. However, in advanced societies, agriculture has become industrialized to the point where both human and animal labor essentially have been replaced by machinery. (Agriculture is addressed in greater detail in subsequent chapters.)

The first farmer still was seminomadic. Poorly productive lands often were quickly exhausted, and farmers moved on to new land. In this way, farming is said to have crept into Europe through the forests. A contemporary example is that of the Iroquois Indians of western New York, who move their villages about every 10 years.

With the adoption of agriculture, populations grew enormously. Land shortages quickly appeared, and the rapid diffusion of the plow was accelerated by major movements of people in search of new lands. Whereas horticulture had diffused slowly into Europe, agriculture virtually swept across the continent.

The Characteristics of Food-producing Societies

Common characteristics of food-producing societies are summarized as follows.

1. Control over the food supply. With the advent of food production, people were able to augment the productivity of the environment, gaining at least some degree of control over their food supply. This circumstance had tremendous ramifications. Fewer people died of malnutrition and disease. Death rates decreased, including infant mortality rates. As a result, populations increased. In many ways, the quality of life increased. (However, some anthropologists and other scholars argue that in some ways the hunting-gathering way of life was superior to one which is agriculturally based.)

2. More sedentary living. While many pastoral people continued to roam with their flocks, others began to raise animals that were better kept in one place. The pig, for example, is notorious for being a poor traveler! And agriculture, of course, necessitated remaining in one place to care for the crops and protect them from marauders. Pastoral people, historically, have been desirous of taking over agricultural fields, since the same land that is used for crops is perceived to be equally suitable for the grazing of pastoral animals.

3. Higher population density.

4. Rise of cities. With the necessity of remaining in one place and the rise of population small groups soon increased to small villages and thence to larger urban centers.

5. More complex political organization. With the increase in the number of people per unit area and the lessened importance of kinship bonds, the need for a more organized government structure evolved.

6. Although there had been some specialization and division of labor within foraging societies, the need for specialists increased greatly with the advent of food production. Various artisans emerged to create the tools needed and used in this more complex society. A host of new inventions came on the heels of expanding agriculture: dairying, the wheel for land transport, the horizontal wheel for pottery turning, and finally, writing and metallurgy.

7. Increase in cultural artifacts. As long as humans lived a nomadic existence, they could not carry many possessions with them. As they became more sedentary, however, they were able to accumulate things they had made, for example, jewelry, works of art, and more tools and clothing. Nomadic people relied exclusively on oral tradition to maintain a history of their past. With the discovery of writing in Mesopotamia about 5,000 years ago, and the growth of sedentary living, mankind began to develop records. The first libraries evolved.

8. The rise of aggression. With more people in one place, tensions increased, and crime as well. Moreover, as Richard Leakey (1981:229) has pointed out, "as soon as people commit themselves to agriculture, they commit themselves to defend the land they farm." He quotes Richard Lee as saying, "When people's livelihood is rooted in the fields, they are imbedded in the land in a way that hunter-gatherers are not." Leakey and Roger Lewin (1977:222–23) attribute the considerable display of aggression on the part of twentieth-century humans to the growth of agriculture and of materially based societies.

9. Need for salt. As humans shifted from a diet high in meat to a grain diet, they

began to ingest larger amounts of potassium, but much less sodium than before. Thus, especially in warm climates where perspiration was profuse, there developed a critical need for an additional source of salt in the diet. This circumstance resulted in the development of the salt trade. Salt became a much coveted commodity, over which many wars have been fought.

10. Rise of civilization. This was the most important factor in the evolution of a society. Foresight and long-range planning became increasingly feasible. Under favorable circumstances, greater leisure was possible, with opportunities for greater creativity and productivity than before.

FOOD PROCESSING

Strictly speaking, food processing is any treatment food undergoes from the time it is produced until it is ingested. The goal of food processing is to improve the quality of food in some way and/or to preserve it. The first foods of humans were raw, obtained by foraging, and were essentially unprocessed. One of the problems that people encountered early in their search for food was that it tended to be perishable. This problem still exists. In fact, the very foods which have the highest nutrient value for humans are also the most perishable (Desrosier 1963:24). Examples are eggs, meat, and milk. Early people often solved the problem of meat spoilage by sharing it after the kill with others. Over time, humans have learned to process food in various ways.

Aging

This process tends to occur spontaneously with meat in the absence of freezing. People found that the changes associated with aging conferred desirable qualities on meat (and a few other foods). In England, for example, poultry and hunted fowl are left to hang out in sheds. As the carcasses age, certain catabolic processes take place, and the pH (degree of acidity or alkalinity) increases. Together, these various changes produce a distinctive flavor, considered pleasing by many. Aged fowl is referred to as "high game," and the flavor is characterized as "high" or "gamey."

Cooking

Involving the application of heat to food, this treatment changes food properties and also aids in food preservation. It is thought to have first consisted of roasting, or broiling. Cooking probably developed shortly after humans learned to use or control fire, about 750,000 years ago at the earliest (Howell 1966; Klein 1979; Gordon 1987:24). Boiling (by pit cooking) is thought to have begun at about 5000 B.C., at the earliest (R. Tannahill 1973:27). Cooking made food more chewable, digestible, and often more palatable. Also, heat killed microorganisms, increasing the keeping qualities of the food. It is widely accepted that the use of fire and the development of containers worked together to make possible the cooking of food. Evidence of meat consumption by early hunters predates the first evidence of fire use by at least 1 million years. So, early phases of cooking may have served mainly to maximize the extent to which meat (and other foods) could be used, rather than enabling man to use previously unexploited food resources (Gordon 1987:25).

Food Preservation

By trial and error, humans learned that there were certain ways of treating foods whereby they could save excess food for use later on. (This is an example of man's developing ability of foresight.)

The earliest form of food preservation was drying—a process that tended to take place automatically, particularly in warm arid climates, where sun and wind both aided in the drying process. In colder climes, an early form of preservation was freezing (which probably tended to occur automatically, as well). The use of salt, either in the pickled (marinated) or dry state, served to dehydrate meat and preserve it. In solutions along with vinegar, it served as a pickling agent in which the food product became dehydrated and most microorganisms could not thrive. Sugar also proved to be a good preservative: it also discouraged microbial growth through its dehydrating effect. When fruit and vegetable juices containing sugar fermented, alcohol, or acid was produced, both of which also discouraged microbial growth. Another fermentation process that benefits human beings is the conversion of chopped green plants to silage, used to feed cattle in winter (Figure 2.4). Corn and sorghum are commonly used for this process.

Two other methods of food preservation (usually for meat) are curing and smoking. Two types of curing are dry curing and curing by use of a pickling solution (Desrosier: 1963:262–64). The ingredients used in curing and pickling are sodium nitrate, sodium nitrite, sodium chloride, sugar, and citric acid (or vinegar). Sugar is used mainly as a flavoring agent in the curing process. Curing can be combined with smoking in preserving animal products. Smoke acts not only as a dehydrating agent, but it deposits a coating on the surface of the meat of materials obtained in the destructive distillation of wood. Small amounts of formaldehyde and other ingredients from the smoke are present and inhibit microbial growth. Smoking thus acts as a preservative complementary to the curing process and also adds flavor to the food product. It probably first occurred inadvertently after the discovery of fire, when animal flesh happened to get too close to the campfire. Both salting and smoking were well established by 1000 B.C.

In addition to certain individual effects, the techniques of drying, pickling, fermentation, salting, smoking, and adding sugar all produce dehy-

Figure 2.4
Old Silo, 1900

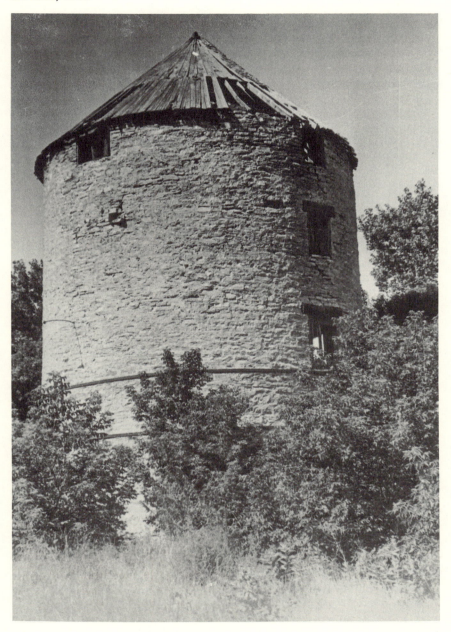

Silos are important for making and preserving silage, which is fed to cattle in winter. Franklin H. King, an agricultural scientist in Wisconsin, built a round silo in 1882. Round silos enable feed to be packed tightly, providing the anaerobic conditions necessary for silage production.

Press Gazette Collection of the Neville Public Museum of Brown County

dration. The latter is a key factor in food preservation, since it discourages microbial growth.

More recently, people have discovered additional techniques such as canning and irradiation. However, these earlier techniques continue to be used.

UNIVERSAL FOODS

As mentioned in the preface, it is important for the student of food habits to develop an awareness of the commonalities among the food habits practiced across time and cultures. Such a nomothetic perspective should prove to be helpful in assessing food habits within specific eras, areas, and cultures. In this section, some of the more salient, recurring commonalities regarding food will be cited.

Making Food Choices

In studying food habits, one is constantly reminded that of necessity human beings always have eaten from what is available. Only from among those foods which are available may people make choices. Further, when allowed a choice, they will tend to adhere to optimal foraging theory. That is, they will choose first from those foods that have the most favorable cost-benefit balances.

In spite of the diversity of man's food habits, there is an amazing commonality across regions and time, with respect to the types of foods and food products used. Undoubtedly, this circumstance has resulted from several factors. First, all human cultures share the same nutritional needs. Second, these needs must be supplied by available foods, and last, these foods tend to fall into predictable categories across the globe.

The general classes of foods chosen by humans, regardless of culture or geographic location, are included in the various food plans that have been released by the federal government. The most recent of these is the Six Food Group Plan (USDA, HNIS 1989), discussed in chapters 1 and 6. Included within these food categories are two foods of unique nutritional significance to people: nuts and honey. Nuts have always been prized. They are nutrient dense and high in calories. So, from the standpoint of optimal foraging theory, it makes sense to gather them. Honey also has been valued by humans, both as a flavorful food and a concentrated form of energy, quickly utilized by the body.

Most persons express surprise that from the large number of foods potentially available, people actually have exploited only a relatively few. Table 2.1 lists the major crops which sustain the world's people today, that is, those produced in amounts of 10 million metric tons or more annually. Of these 29 crops, there are 9 with annual harvests of over 100 million metric tons. Together, these 9 crops produce over three and a half times

Table 2.1
Major Food Crops of the World

Crop	Production[1]
Wheat[2]	595
Rice[2]	519
Maize[2]	475
Potato[3]	301
Barley	177
Cassava	136
Sweet potato	111
Millet and sorghum	105
Soybeans	101
Sugarcane	96
Tomatoes	60
Grapes	60
Oats	50
Coconut	41
Banana	40
Sugar beet	39
Apples	38
Cabbages	38
Oranges	38
Rye	33
Cottonseed	33
Watermelon	28
Onions, dry	24
Groundnuts (peanuts)	21
Sunflower seed	19
Rapeseed	19
Beans, dry	15
Peas, dry	13
Pineapple	10

[1]Expressed as millions of metric tons.

[2]1990 values. FAO 1994.

[3]Potatoes and ensuing crops: 1985 values. FAO 1987.

the tonnage of the remaining 20. Similarly, most of the world's meat comes from only four categories of animals (Table 2.2). The most commonly consumed meat is pork, followed by beef (and small amounts of buffalo). Poultry consumption is third, with mutton a distant fourth in terms of consumption (Food and Agriculture Organization [FAO] 1987).

As food foragers, humans are thought to have used several thousand species of plants and several hundred species of animals. However, with the beginnings of agriculture, only a relatively small number of these species were ever domesticated (Harlan, 1976). There was a tendency to concen-

Table 2.2
World Meat Production

Meat	Production[1]
Pork	59
Beef and buffalo	48
Poultry	31
Mutton	8

[1]Expressed as millions of metric tons.
Source: FAO 1987.

trate on those species which were most rewarding in terms of labor and capital investment. This behavior also supports the optimal foraging theory.

Even the modern day hunter-gatherers, the !Kung Bushmen of the Kalahari Desert in Africa, obtain 90 percent of their diet by weight from 23 species of edible plants, including the very popular mongongo, baobab, and marula nuts (Lee 1972:25).

The trend for more and more people to be nourished by fewer and fewer plant and animal food sources has reached the point today where most of the world's people are absolutely dependent on a handful of species. The crops most in demand are wheat, rice, maize, and the potato, in descending order (Table 2.1).

It is noteworthy that the major crops listed in Table 2.1 include the "sacred grains"—the seven prime grains that have been pivotal in sustaining human beings for at least 10,000 years, since the beginning of the Neolithic period (Figure 2.1). Of the seven, wheat, rice, barley, oats, and millet were the first ones domesticated in the Old World. Rye assumed importance after the ebbing of the Greek and Roman civilizations, particularly in Europe. Historically, maize is the indigenous staple of the Western Hemisphere. It spread to the Old World when it was brought by the Portuguese to the Congo and Angola from Brazil in the sixteenth century (Crosby 1972:187).

Predictable Food Products

In handling food materials, most cultures have become aware of the advantages of certain techniques or processes whereby the keeping quality, palatability, and/or other desired properties were enhanced. These considerations undoubtedly have influenced the development of predictable types of food products, or universal foods, which have endured through time and across cultures. Some examples of these universal foods are shown in Table 2.3.

Pasta products. Many cultures have found that grinding cereals and other

Table 2.3
Universal Food Products

General Category	Examples
Soft cheeses	Cream, cottage, feta, ricotta
Leavened breads	Rolls, biscuits, loaf breads
Unleavened breads, soft, thin	Lefse, tortillas
Unleavened breads, crisp, thin	Flat breads, matzos, tostados
Fermented products	Hard cheeses, pickled fruits and vegetables, some sausages, alcoholic beverages
Pastas	Noodles, macaroni, fettucine, lasagna
Blood products	Blood soup, blood sausage (klub)
Sauces, gravies	Vegetable or meat stocks, or milk, thickened with flour, starch, powdered sassafras, or okra
Sausages	Meat, ground with added spices, chopped cabbage, cheese, or other condiments
Dried meat products	Jerky; pemmican

starchy foods to make some type of flour, adding water to make a paste, then air drying, heating, or boiling the paste provides the foundation for many kinds of "pasta" products. Examples include noodles, lasagna, macaroni, spaghetti, and dumplings. The noodle is thought to have originated in China.

Fermented foods and beverages. Leaving things out in the open attracted yeasts and other microbes which fed on certain foods, especially those with an appreciable sugar content. During the metabolism of the microbes feeding on these foods, certain products were produced that often increased their palatability and, almost always, their keeping qualities, as well. Many of these processes occurred spontaneously. But as the desirability of these products began to be recognized, conditions conducive to selected fermentations deliberately were encouraged and controlled.

Many food products are the result of fermentations of fruits, vegetables, meat, and milk, and cereals. They include pickled foods, wines, sausages, cheeses, and breads.

Since fermentations often occur spontaneously, every culture, beginning in the earliest of times, has discovered and learned to prize alcoholic beverages that have resulted from the fermentation of sugar-containing foods. Not only was the taste of the product usually pleasant, there were certain euphoric effects as well. These psychological effects were recognized early (Proverbs 31:6–7)—and constitute a universal human experience. Alcoholic beverages have been produced from the fermentation of such diverse sugar-containing foods as grapes, dates, palm, sugarcane, animal milks, and honey (mead).

Certain types of soft white cheese, produced by a basic lactic acid fermentation are produced universally. They include cream, cottage, feta, and ricotta cheeses.

Breads. Another food genre from cereals and other starchy products are breads, both leavened and unleavened. Leavened bread products have a soft, fluffy texture due to bubbles of carbon dioxide produced by a yeast fermentation or the action of baking powder. These bubbles escape during the baking process, altering texture. Unleavened breads contain little or no leavening agent and usually are rolled out or pressed until thin. They may be baked briefly, yielding a soft, doughy product (e.g., lefse, rieska, and tortillas), or baked and/or fried until crisp (e.g., flat breads, tostados, and matzos).

It is difficult, if not impossible, to determine with certainty which peoples discovered which products first, since so many of these processes probably occurred spontaneously under the right conditions, throughout the world.

REVOLUTIONARY EVENTS IN HISTORY

Important events in history which greatly altered the way people live (including their food habits) include:

1. The beginnings of culture: bipedalism, communication, the first tools, the use and control of fire.

2. The development of food production.

3. The development of metallurgy.

4. Urbanization and specialization.

5. The industrial revolution: the application of mechanical power to the processes of production; the development of scientific methods.

6. The postindustrial era: the age of biotechnology (see chapters 6 and 10).

FOR FURTHER READING

Beals, R.L., and H. Hoijer. 1971. *An introduction to anthropology* (4th ed.). New York: Macmillan Company.

Dahlberg, F. 1981. Introduction. In F. Dahlberg (ed.), *Woman the gatherer* (1–33). New Haven, CT: Yale University Press.

Gordon, K.E. 1987. Evolutionary perspectives in human diet. In F.E. Johnston (ed.), *Nutritional anthropology* (3–39). New York: Alan R. Liss.

Harlan, J.R. 1976. The plants and animals that nourish man. *Scientific American* 235(3): 88–97.

Harris, M., and E.B. Ross. 1987. *Food and evolution*. Philadelphia: Temple University Press.

Johnston, F.E. (ed.). 1987. *Nutritional anthropology*. New York: Alan R. Liss.

Leakey, R.E. 1981. *The making of mankind*. New York: E.P. Dutton.

Lee, R.B. 1972. *The !Kung San*. Cambridge: Cambridge University Press.

Lee, R.B., and I. deVore. 1968. *Man the hunter*. Chicago: Aldine.

Tannahilll, R. 1973. *Food in history*. New York: Stein and Day.

Figure 3.1
Paleo-Indian Slays Wounded Mastodon

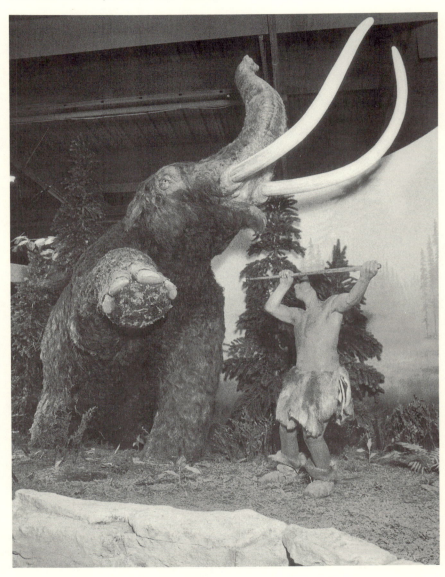

The Neville Public Museum of Brown County

3

Early Dietary Patterns

This chapter is concerned with the evolution of food habits from primitive times through the Middle Ages, chiefly emphasizing Europe and North America. Its focus is how the ancestors of post-Columbian North Americans ate. In addition to its being of intrinsic interest, this information should be helpful in gaining an understanding of American food practices, from post-Columbian times through the present.

THE EASTERN HEMISPHERE

Food Gathering

Modern Homo sapiens evolved from Homo erectus, an advanced hominid who lived 1.5 million years ago to 300,000 years ago. Originating in Africa, these early humans were the first people to migrate from that continent, eventually reaching northern Asia and Europe.

Homo erectus is thought to be the first human to use and control fire, dating to about 750,000 years ago (Bonifay and Bonifay 1963; Howell 1966; Klein 1979). The mastery of fire would have served several important purposes. Fire could be used to drive game, to keep predators at bay, to provide warmth, and to aid in food preparation, storage, and preservation. These early people also were the first humans to use stone tools (e.g., a crude ax). Superior tools, coupled with a larger brain and body size and more efficient bipedalism, enabled Homo erectus to develop specialized hunting and other food-gathering techniques. These activities were continued and perfected through the end of the Pleistocene (and beyond) by Homo sapiens (chapter 1).

About 250,000 years ago, Homo erectus began evolving into Homo sapiens, the earliest examples of which have been found in England and Germany. Remains of a somewhat later type, the Neanderthal, also have been found. Neanderthal man lived in parts of Africa, Asia, and Europe from about 100,0000 to 35,000 years ago. Their brains were as large as those of modern human beings. On the basis of fossil evidence, modern human beings began to appear about 40,000 years ago. The best-known early form of modern human being is the Cro-Magnon, who lived in northern Africa, western and central Asia, and Europe. Both the Neanderthals and Cro-Magnons made flake tools, fished, and hunted birds and large game (Butzer 1989:15,755). The evolution of Homo sapiens occurred at different times in different parts of the world, probably first in Africa and Europe and much later in eastern Asia (754).

Food Production

The end of the glacial period marked a shift in emphasis by various human populations from hunting and gathering to more intense control over plants and animal resources through domestication (Gordon 1987:3–4). During their early shift toward food production, early peoples living in what is now Europe were much influenced by the advances of four great earlier civilizations, which had emerged in Africa and Asia.

Sumer (Mesopotamia). About 3500 B.C., (5,500 years ago) the Sumerians began to build the world's first culture and its first civilization in Mesopotamia, between the Tigris and Euphrates rivers. The earliest use of bronze also occurred there.

Egypt. Another advanced culture arose relatively soon after, in Egypt, along the Nile Valley, about 3000 B.C. (5,000 years ago). It flourished for over 2,000 years, one of the longest-lasting civilizations in history.

The Indus Valley. A third ancient civilization developed along the Indus River, in what is now Pakistan and the Punjab area in northwestern India. It thrived about 2500 B.C. (4,500 years ago).

The Huang He Valley. A fourth great civilization arose along the banks of the Huang He (Yellow) River before 2000 B.C. (see Jensen 1953:56 for details). Here animal husbandry was practiced, and rice and millet were grown as staple foods.

These four early civilizations all developed along rivers, a typical pattern, historically, the world over. All of these areas undoubtedly began their food production as horticulturists, or as incipient agriculturists. Animal husbandry probably developed at the same time. The arid conditions brought

Table 3.1
The Development of Metallurgy

Metal or Alloy	Near East	Europe	North America
Bronze	Before 3500 B.C.	1900–1800 B.C. (Central Europe) 1500 B.C. (Scandinavian Peninsula)	———
Iron	1500 B.C. Anatolian Plateau	750 B.C. (Central Europe) Before 400 B.C. (England and Scandinavia)	17th century: arrival of British colonists
Steel	300 B.C. Eastern Africa (small amounts)	Middle Ages (small amounts) Crucible Process: 1740 (Britain)	1748

Source: R.L. Beals and H. Hoijer 1971:301–302; D. Beaver 1989: vol. 10, 451.

both man and animals closer together, as they gathered around water sources (e.g., along the Nile, in Egypt). This situation encouraged the domestication of animals. Moreover, the extinction of large game may have encouraged man to tame and care for smaller animals during this general period. Pastoralism undoubtedly developed in those climates or areas where animals could not be fed in closed quarters. Although it served as a means whereby people could support flocks, pastoralism necessitated at least a seasonal nomadism. Seasonal nomadism still can be observed in several parts of the world today, for example, Afghanistan, Lapland, Norway, and Alaska.

Metallurgy. With the development of metallurgy (Table 3.1), the early societies could fashion not only jewelry, but important tools and weapons for improving both their hunting and fishing and pots for roasting and baking. Further, it provided tools for raising crops on a larger scale, enabling the transition from horticulture to agriculture.

The early Neolithic people used weapons and tools of wood and stone. The Bronze Age is that period within the late Neolithic when copper and bronze (an alloy of 25 percent tin and 75 percent copper) began to replace such assemblages. The Bronze Age began at different times, depending on the area, and ended with the beginning of the Iron Age (Table 3.1). In most places, the Bronze Age overlapped the Stone Age, and also a later Iron Age, because people did not stop using one material all at once. For example, during the Bronze Age, most artisans continued to use stone tools, for metal was expensive. The use of iron was a significant advance, since it was stronger than bronze; it also was more abundant and widespread, and, hence, cheaper. People learned early that iron became even stronger when it was mixed with small amounts of other elements, such as carbon and manganese. Thus steelmaking began.

Ancient Greece

The Greek civilization, which followed the great civilizations described above, was the first great culture to originate on the European continent. It began to develop about 2000 B.C. and peaked in Athens during the period known as the Golden Age (477–431 B.C.). During this time, the Greeks made high attainments in philosophy, the arts, trade, and in the development of a democratic government. The influence of ancient Greece went far beyond its borders; in fact, it today is regarded as the birthplace of Western civilization.

The Athenians made all of their products by hand. They were famous for their pottery. The ancient Greeks also made armor and clothing. Corinth was noted for jewelry and metal goods (e.g., bronze helmets), about 550–500 B.C.—just before the Golden Age. The world's best-known temples were built on the Acropolis, during the 400s B.C.

Food supply. Agriculture in Greece was well over 1,000 years behind that of Mesopotamia and Egypt. According to Homer, the Greek poet (800–700 B.C.?), animal husbandry was still the main source of subsistence in 1000 B.C. The warriors of Greece in the twelfth century B.C. were descendants of the nomadic pastoralists of Central Asia and probably had retained a similar lifestyle (Tannahill 1973:71).

By about 2000 B.C., people from someplace to the north came down and began to establish small farming villages. By the 700s B.C., the Greek world consisted of many small independent city-states. The most fertile land was in the small villages and along the coast; much of Greece, however, was covered by rocky, light soil. Nevertheless, as long as the population remained small, the people were able to eke out a modest food supply.

Diets in early Greece. The early Greek diet was simple. Porridge and bread from wheat and barley were eaten, olives, olive oil, some fish, figs, honey, cheese, and wine. Peasant families usually kept a goat for milk and cheese, and, occasionally, some pigs. The richer farmer might have a flock of sheep. However, since Greece's thin, arid soil did not lend itself to much stock raising, meat tended to be scarce, and was used mainly for feasts and at times of religious sacrifices. Like the Egyptians and Romans, the Greeks rarely drank milk, but they did make cheese—usually of the feta type.

Most Greeks were largely vegetarians. Common foods included beans, cabbage, leeks, lentils, onions, turnips, and some fruits. The Greek diet emphasized porridges or grain pastes (maza), usually made from barley or lentils. The city-state of Sparta was known for its "black broth," made from pork stock, blood, vinegar and salt.

Problems of food and agriculture. As the population increased, there was increased competition for the small amount of available land, which had to be used more intensively. It suffered from overuse by sheep, whose grazing habits left the ground almost bare, and from overcropping. For several reasons, the people were forced into clearing much of the remaining tree-covered land. Wood was needed for shelter and ships and for charcoal to use in metal working. Moreover, the cleared land provided new fields for the raising of more food for the rising, hungry population. Thus, sheep grazing, overcropping, and removal of trees all increased the erosion of the already vulnerable, light, dry, Grecian soil. In addition, the dry, warm climate encouraged the buildup of salinity in the soil, thus discouraging the growth of many crops. Under these conditions, the Greek landscape became bleak (Burn 1967:67–68). The beloved meadows, woods, and springs of the past disappeared, a state of affairs lamented by Plato (Coon 1954:293).

Fortunately, olives, grapevines, and barley tolerated high salt content and aridity well. The olive, followed by wine, became the two chief exports of Greece by about the sixth century B.C. Olives and grapes (along with fig and nut trees) took over, at the expense of livestock, barley, and wheat. Importation became a virtual necessity, to ensure an adequate food supply.

The Golden Age: A dichotomy of diets. Until the middle of the fifth century B.C., the diet of the rich and poor in Greece probably did not differ greatly. Because of the polluted water, the rich may have drunk more wine than the peasants and may also have eaten meat and game more often. However, by the time Athens was at its height, there was a great disparity between rich and poor cuisine (Tannahill 1973:82). While poor Athenians ate black pudding made from blood, the rich dined on exotic foods available through importation. The Greeks began to produce cookbooks in the fourth century B.C. (Lowenberg et al. 1979:31).

Grecian wines. Between 500 and 100 B.C., Greece was famous in the Mediterranean world for its fine wines, but the Greek cuisine never approached that of the French. The rich of the Mediterranean countries liked imported wines, especially those from two Greek islands in the Aegean Sea, Lesbos and Chios (the latter the home of Chianti). They also liked sweet wines (e.g., the Pramnian of Homer, and mead, from honey and herbs). The Greeks (and Romans) followed the Egyptian custom of diluting wine with water, to dilute the salt used in wine as a preservative at that time. This practice also resulted in a beverage with a sharply reduced alcohol content.

Decline of Athens. The Golden Age ended with the outbreak of the Peloponnesian War in 431 B.C. between Athens and Sparta. In 430 B.C., a severe plague hit Athens, killing about a third of the population. The decline of Athens after 350 B.C. was closely associated with food shortages caused by the lack of exports and, subsequently, a lack of money, to import needed foods. The Romans took over Greece and Macedonia in the 140s B.C.

The Peloponnesian wars during the latter part of the fifth century were devastating to the Attic countryside. Villages were razed, and crops were ruined. Recovery was slow and difficult, especially because of the length of time required for the maturation of new olive trees (30 years) and vines (3 to 4 years) (Tannahill 1973). Peasants sold out and moved to the city.

The wreckage caused by these wars served to exacerbate the serious problems already faced by Greek agriculture. At the same time, a still rising population meant increasing demands for food. More crops were needed to supply food at home. All of these factors led to a marked reduction in exportable goods by which to obtain imported food in return.

Return to austere diets. Faced with food scarcity, Athenians were forced to return to a drab diet: cooked cereal with figs and dried dates, or olives and cheese. The staple was bread with oil, wine, or honey.

Summary. Overall, the Grecian life was rather sparse. There was a lack of technology, even little use of animals as beasts of burden. The Greek philosophers stopped with theory. Beginning with little data, they developed their theories by the application of logic but failed to translate them into practice. The decline of Athens, after 350 B.C., and the later decline of the Roman Empire, after A.D. 476, occurred when there were food shortages; exports had fallen, and there was no money for imported food. As with most civilizations, their fates were closely tied to their food supplies.

Ancient Rome

The earliest evidences of habitation in this area of Europe date back to about 1500 B.C., when invaders from Central Europe settled in the Po Valley. Judging from bronze objects that have been found, these people were already familiar with the use of that alloy. Villages unearthed in the 1880s showed that they established villages and absorbed and dominated the existing Neolithic peoples. By 900–800 B.C., the Etruscans, a later group of invaders, had appeared, and were living north of the Tiber. They are thought to have been traders who came from Asia Minor, probably in search of copper and tin for their bronze industry. Bringing an advanced culture with them, they endured long enough to leave a lasting mark on Roman civilization. The Etruscan society was one of distinct upper and lower classes. Each of their cities was ruled by priest kings (Lowenberg et al. 1979:33). They built a wall around Rome, drained swamps, and laid the first sewer (in evidence yet today).

Rome had been a simple farming community until 600 B.C., when it came under the control of the Etruscans. At the beginning of its history, a series of kings had ruled Rome. Then in 509 B.C., the Roman nobles overthrew the monarchy and established a republic. The Appian Way was built in 312 B.C., during this period. By 270 B.C., the Romans had conquered the Greek cities in Italy and Sicily and had unified the entire southern peninsula into a single alliance. Under Etruscan rule during the 500s B.C. Rome grew from a village to a city. In 27 B.C., the Roman Empire was established, following 20 years of civil war that had destroyed the Republic. The Empire lasted until the fall of Rome in A.D. 476.

Food patterns during the Republic. Up through the second century B.C., the Romans ate frugally. They were vegetarians, eating their food cold. Their utensils were modest, with one exception: a penchant for the silver salt shaker. Salt was considered a necessity at table, and the honored place was "to be seated above the salt." Bread was such a staple in the Roman diet that the word became synonymous with the word food (as it is in the Bible) (Lowenberg et al.:37). Bread often was used as a "mop," since dishes were not commonly used. There was yet little distinction among the classes.

When Rome defeated Carthage in North Africa in the second century B.C., it gained control of the wheat of Egypt, North Africa, and Sicily. These and other successful conquests during the last two centuries of the Republic led to vastly improved living conditions for the rich. The importation of food from Mesopotamia, north Africa, and elsewhere, provided new dietary possibilities for members of the new upper class. Meat and fish became easily available. Wine was drunk primarily by the upper classes, usually diluted 8:1, as the Greeks did, to reduce the salt content. The Romans admired the Greek culture greatly and sought to emulate it as much as possible, including its food habits. However, they became gluttons, rather than gourmets, as were the elite in Greece. Nevertheless, by 121 B.C., they had begun to surpass the Greeks with respect to their reputation for fine wines.

Meanwhile, the poor Romans continued to eat simply. Their diet consisted mainly of a polentalike porridge made from millet, grain pastes, coarse bread, olive oil and water. In addition, turnips, olives, beans, figs, and cheese were available (Tannahill 1973). Meat was scarce, except for an occasional pig or some fish (for those who lived close to water). Because of primitive cooking facilities, lack of fuel, and the risk of fire in the crowded tenement houses, the poor avoided cooking as much as possible (Carcopino 1940:30).

Food habits during the Roman Empire. This period began in 27 B.C. Roman rule first spread slowly over all the lands bordering the Mediterranean Sea. But by A.D. 9, the Romans had overtaken Germany and were planting their grapevines on the steep slopes of the Rhine Valley, as well as in the Holy Land. At its maximum size in the 100s A.D., the Roman Empire extended as far north as the British Isles and as far east as the Persian Gulf. Almost every known food now was available through importation from somewhere within this vast domain. While poor Romans continued to eat simply, as they always had, affluent Romans became even more engrossed than ever in the pleasures of food and drink. Wealthy Romans devoted much time and money on banquets and dinner parties. For a full dinner party, the Romans preferred nine people, compared to the Greeks, who preferred five. Nine guests customarily reclined on three couches arranged in a U shape around a table. They reclined at three-quarter length on their left arm, eating with their right fingers (Nero fashion!).

Downfall of Roman Empire, A.D. 476. By the beginning of the fifth century A.D., the ruling upper-class Romans had become attached to a life of pleasure, luxury, and sensual gratification. They were in no frame of mind to cope with the hardships and problems of conquest nor with the administration of lands which their conquests had brought them. At the same time, they had become weakened by the repeated onslaughts of the Germanic tribes from the north, which had persisted for centuries. Now, the Germans had appeared outside the gates of the city again. By A.D. 476, Odoacer (their chieftain) had deposed Romulus Augustus, the last Roman emperor in the west.

Cities were a natural magnet for invaders, forcing the townspeople to relocate in the countryside. Exodus from city to land occurred. Until the Industrial Revolution, 90 percent of the population was engaged in agriculture, constituting the "silent majority" (even during urbanized times) (White 1962:39).

The German barbarians disrupted political unity. Currency crises forced a return to a barter economy. Imported goods were being sold at prices lower than domestically produced food. Finally, disintegration of the empire led to dislocation of such organized trade as survived. The final downfall of the great Roman Empire had occurred.

Middle Ages in Europe

Crop failures and famine. The Middle Ages are sometimes called the Years of Famine, because of the poor crops and scarcity of food that characterized this period (A.D. 476–1500). During the Early Middle Ages, agriculture was besieged by diseases (especially ergotism and black stem rust), which ruined crops and seriously reduced the amount of available food. Ergotism also caused violent convulsions, abortions in pregnant women, and, frequently, deaths. While the entire period between the eighth and fourteenth century has been characterized as bad, the ninth and tenth centuries in northern and western Europe were especially plagued by famines (Walford 1879; Tannahill 1973:116–18).

As in all ages, bread had been the standby and a favorite food of all. So when the grain failed, because of poor agricultural methods, the Crusades, drought, or disease, people starved. People resorted to the acorn in times of famine, especially in France. They had lived on the oak tree's acorn before the era of grain. Acorn bread was better than that which the Germans made from grass, seeds, and roots. Man was turning back thousands of years to the food-gathering period by reverting to the acorn. The most unnatural breads ever baked came from Sweden in these times; they were 90 percent bark and straw. Baking dried meat blood with flour was revived wherever animals were available (e.g., Norwegian "klub"). Unfortunately, some people resorted to cannibalism.

These bleak years of famine are reflected in the nursery rhymes, which despite controversies regarding their origin, graphically depict the scarcity of, and subsequent preoccupation with, food during that period. Medieval art also provides one with insight into the food habits of the period.

Food habits. During the early medieval period, food was cooked using fires in the center of the hut. Pollution was rampant. One-dish meals were prepared in "cauldrons," or kettles, suspended on a spit over the fire. These pots simmered all day and rarely were cleaned out, as implied in the well-known nursery rhyme "Pease Porridge Hot."

Rye became the principal cereal grown in northern and western Europe. It was the hardiest of all cereals and was favored by the Teutonic tribesmen. Thus, the everyday bread of the Middle Ages was "pumpernickel," made from rye. Unlike wheat, rye does not contain enough glutenin and gliadin to make well-risen bread. So the bread of the Middle Ages was rather heavy. When wheat was available, it was often made into frumenty. Made by soaking the husked grains in hot water for twenty-four hours, it was eaten with milk and honey.

Common staples were bread, ale, and salt pork. Except for cabbage, leeks and onions, vegetables were scarce or absent from the diet during this period. The food supply was markedly seasonal. There was a barren period in the last months of winter, when fresh foods were especially lacking. Fainting was common amongst women, caused by anemia—frequent child bearing and the result of lack of dietary iron.

A serf of the eighth century produced his own wine and raised pigs, calves, chickens, and eggs on his plot of land. Wild game occasionally appeared on his table, but fruit was rare. The usual foods were bread, ale, salt pork, stewed cabbage, and root crops.

Feudal barons, on the other hand, dined on a variety of meats, mammoth roasts, wild boar, venison, veal, game, ducks, geese, and chicken. They would also have fish, if they lived near a sea, lake, or river. Bread, cheese, and honey commonly were available. However, the meat, cheese, and bread diet became monotonous. Spices were eagerly sought in order to camouflage the tainted meat and liven up the diet.

Early Middle Ages (fifth through the tenth centuries). After the fall of Rome, imported foods became almost nonexistent, throughout inland and northern Europe, especially. Most people were forced again to rely on foods from their immediate area.

Teutonic tribesmen adopted the Roman habit of using slaves for farming. Disliking hard labor and agriculture, they made slaves of the descendants of enslaved Roman colonists ("serfs"). Paganism and Christianity battled side by side over control of the farmland. The barbarians wanted to leave everything to nature, and not cultivate the soil. But the monks refused to do this. The Romans at this time possessed great agricultural knowledge, including familiarity with crop rotation, irrigation, tools, fertilizers. But it was difficult to impart this knowledge to the invaders because of the language barrier. In addition, the agricultural literature was in Latin. However, in spite of these obstacles, frequent crop failures, and famine, the monks (who were among the few people literate in Latin or any other language) during the Middle Ages had an important influence on the development of agriculture all through Europe.

The Saracens invaded Spain from North Africa during the 700s; a positive aspect of their conquest was that it initiated a period of market gardening. Bringing sugar cane and rice with them, along with other important cultivated plants, they introduced many new foods to Europe. Moorish Spain became noted for its agriculture.

*High Middle Ages (*A.D. *1050–1300).* This period was marked by the Crusades, a series of eight major Christian military expeditions between A.D. 1096 and 1270, aimed ostensibly at gaining permanent control of the Holy Land and to protect the Byzantine Empire. However, many crusaders also sought increased power, land, and wealth. John Elson (1992:19) has described these mixed motives as "religious zeal blended uneasily with unabashed greed." The Crusades to recover the Holy Land during the eleventh, twelveth, and thirteenth centuries were bad for agriculture in Europe. The men were gone, and the farming was left to the women, children, and older men, who were left behind. From the tenth to the fifteenth century, the best of agriculture in Europe moved from Spain to Northern Italy and from there to the Netherlands.

*Late Middle Ages (*A.D. *1300–1500).* By about 1300, Europe experienced a depression in the aftermath of the debilitating wars of previous centuries. The Black Death (bubonic plague) between 1348–49 was even more devastating, killing off a quarter of Europe's population. But despite these hardships, this period also marked the beginning of the Renaissance ("rebirth"). It originated in Italy and spread through Europe. During the Dark Ages, after the fall of Rome, and through the thirteenth century, there had been little emphasis on learning and scientific endeavor. The energies of Western Europeans had been focused on the spread of Christianity and the Crusades (aimed at recapturing the Holy Land). But with the Renaissance came a revival of learning. During the Late Middle Ages, Europe had come a long way with respect to increased maritime prowess, making longer and more frequent voyages possible. By the 1400s, affluent Europeans were very much interested in various types of imported goods: jewels, porcelain, silk, and rare spices. But animosity between Christendom and Islam in the Middle East had resulted in Europeans being cut off from land routes to India and China. Therefore, they were in need of new avenues of trade with the Far East to obtain these coveted items (Elson 1992:19). In addition, population increases had sparked interest in exploiting new lands for colonization, to produce goods and serve as an area to resettle the overflow of population. All of these pressures made exploration increasingly attractive. The stage was set for the Age of European Exploration.

WESTERN HEMISPHERE

The Earliest Immigrants

During the late Pleistocene, at least 20,000 years ago, when the Bering Straits became dry land, people began to cross over from Siberia into what is now Alaska. They were not Mongoloids, but probably people who were the common ancestors of the present-day Chinese and Japanese, and of the American Indian. Because the climate of Siberia was harsh, it is unlikely that many people lived near the Bering land bridge. Consequently, these early immigrants and those who followed them must have been few in number, as well (Crosby 1972:23,30).

These early Asian newcomers were a fully developed form of Homo sapiens. Yet, they appear to have lacked tools, and they certainly had not yet taken up agriculture. With the possible exception of the dog (Zeuner 1963: 436–39), they also must have been unfamiliar with the domestication of animals. They came at a time that long predated the first Sumerian city and long before the Chinese had begun to write (Crosby 1972:31). Some time after the crossing of these early Asian people into North America, the Bering Straits became submerged again, cutting off Asia from North America for a long period. Thus, the American Indians evolved in complete isolation, a circumstance which has rendered them different from the rest of mankind in a number of important ways. Having lived in the harsh environment of Siberia, and then in the northern latitudes of North America, where only the fittest survived, they had evolved into strong human beings. But, at the same time, the members of this group were vulnerable to the new diseases brought in by Columbus and other Europeans (30–31).

The first arrivals must have been food foragers, who searched for plant and animal foods without the aid of special technology. Mainly, they probably subsisted on whatever plant foods were available in the Alaskan climate, augmented by bird eggs and occasional small animals that could be caught with the hands. Less often, they may have exploited larger animals who had been maimed or who had died. It is believed that they and their descendants, the Paleo-Indians, continued to use this most rudimentary method of obtaining food for several thousand years.

The Paleo-Indian Period (13000–8000 B.C.)

During this period, big game was plentiful in North America, and hunting opportunities must have been splendid. Unfortunately, since the Indians did not yet have tools, their ability to exploit this attractive food resource had to have been limited. Instead, they are thought to have continued with their original foraging activities for subsistence.

But, somewhere about 10000 B.C., or before, these descendants of the immigrant foragers became hunter-collectors who had learned to make tools and missile weapons (Figure 3.1). Massive spearheads dating to this period have been found near Clovis, New Mexico, among the bone remains of mammoths, American camels, and hairy elephants. Such instruments enabled them to obtain vastly more meat in the form of the large animals roaming the grasslands during this pre-Boreal period (Dort and Jones 1970). These large herd animals included extinct forms of bison and mammoth. Bison was the primary game animal (Wedel 1961). With tools, the Indians also could collect plant foods more efficiently. These advances made for a better, more dependable food supply.

With the dry climate and plentiful meat supply, game became the dietary staple. Hearths and charred bones excavated in Fort Collins, Colorado, indicate that at least some portions of the meat was cooked (Jennings 1968).

Indians of this period used simple technology for killing game. Native materials such as flint and obsidian were used in the manufacture of large points, which were attached to the end of wooden shafts to form spears (Jerome 1981:38).

Archaic Indian Period (8000–1500 B.C.)

At the beginning of this period, the Indians were continuing to practice both hunting and collecting, that is, obtaining both animal and plant foods using special techniques. Nutritional adequacy must have been generally good. However, after the end of the Ice Age, and the glacial retreat, the climate became hot and dry. The grasslands disappeared, and except in the extreme Southeast portion of the United States, large animals of the Pleistocene became extinct (Krieger 1964:23). The disappearing grasslands, upon which the large animals depended for sustenance, led to a sharp reduction in their numbers, which, in turn, led to overkilling. These two circumstances, together, eventually led to their extinction. The Indians now were forced to hunt smaller animals, providing much lesser quantities of meat. Fortunately, the new Boreal climate favored the growth of plants, upon which, through necessity, the Indians became increasingly dependent for their daily diet. As a result, collecting, as a food-getting activity, was stimulated. It is not surprising that grinding implements (manos and metates) appeared during this Archaic Period. Staple plants used during this time included beans, corn, acorns and chestnuts; however, they were not cultivated (Jerome 1981:38). But, because of this intensive use of collected plant materials, conditions now were favorable for the development of horticulture, which is thought to have emerged in North America during this epoch.

The absence of large game animals and increased availability of plants led to a more sedentary lifestyle (Griffin 1964).

Woodland Indians Period (1500 B.C.–A.D. 300)

Plant domestication and horticulture became intensively used during this era, leading to the real beginning of agriculture (albeit on a small scale). The Woodlands people lived in small villages near water sources and are believed to have been the first truly sedentary people in America. Their sedentary lifestyle is thought to have arisen from two innovations: the development of the storage pit and the development of pottery (Wedel 1964: 193). The storage pit usually was a bell-shaped hole dug in the ground and lined with grass. It served to store grains and nuts that were gathered. Pottery facilitated the storage and transportation of water and enabled meats and grains to be cooked by methods other than roasting. (Jerome 1981:38).

The ability to store food has been a significant breakthrough in the development of every society. For the Woodland Indian, it meant that less time was needed for food gathering, allowing more time for agriculture. The Woodland Period marks the true beginnings of agricultural food production and food storage in the area now known as the United States.

In addition to food crops, game animals and shellfish continued to be important components of the Woodland diet (Sears 1964:259). Small game animals also were utilized. Two new weapons were developed: the bow and arrow and the blow dart (Jennings 1964). The hoe also emerged, providing technological evidence for the domestication of plants during this epoch. In the Great Plains region, the hoe was made from the scapula of a bison (Wedel 1961), whereas in the Southeast, the hoe was made from a mussel shell (Sears 1964). Carbonized remains dating from 1000 B.C. show that a number of plants were domesticated. In the Northeast, these included corn, chenopodium, gourds, marshelder and sunflowers (Griffin 1964:223). The more elaborate technology which appeared during this epoch had a significant impact on the physical and social environment, and subsequently, on the food system and dietary patterns (Jerome 1981:38).

Mississippian Indian Period (A.D. 300–1500)

The presence of dwelling units and villages dating to this period is indicative of an advanced social environment, with increased interaction among the Mississippian Indians. There also are indications of religious life and the beginning of intensive agriculture. These people settled in fertile river valley areas, conducive to the raising and domestication of plants. Staple crops now were maize, beans, pumpkins, and squash. Hoes, spades, and plowing equipment were used by this group (Wedel 1964). Thus, this period is viewed as marking the beginnings of intensive agriculture in North America.

In addition to crop raising, hunting and fishing remained important, as well as collecting. The latter activity provided fruits, roots and berries, which lent variety to this diet (Cassidy 1980).

The Arrival of the Europeans

By the time the Europeans began to arrive, the North American Indians had diffused both southward and eastward, into Central and South America, to Eastern North America and the Caribbean. At the time of Columbus's landfall, the Indians, both in the West Indies and on the North American continent, were well into the latter part of the Mississippian period. Although their agriculture was impressive, they had few domesticated animals: mainly, the dog, the turkey, and the duck. The Indians were without horses, since the latter had long been extinct in America. Barely out of the Stone Age, their bows and arrows could not compete with the Europeans' muskets (Crosby 1972:21,35).

FOR FURTHER READING

Black, M. 1992. *The medieval cookbook.* New York: Thames and Hudson, Inc.

Burn, A.R. 1967. *A traveller's history of Greece.* New York: Funk and Wagnall.

Carcopino, J. 1940. *Daily life in ancient Rome: the people and the city at the height of the Empire.* New Haven, CT: Yale University Press.

Cassidy, C.M. 1980. Nutrition and health in agriculturists and hunter-gatherers: a case study of two prehistoric populations. In N.W. Jerome, R.F. Kandel, and G.H. Pelto (eds.), *Nutritional anthropology* (117–145). Pleasantville, NY: Redgrave Publishing Company.

Gordon, K.D. 1987. Evolutionary perspectives on human diet. In F.E. Johnston (ed.), *Nutritional anthropology* (3–39). New York: Alan R. Liss.

Jennings, E.D., and E. Norbeck (eds.) 1964. *Prehistoric man in the New World* (6th ed.). Chicago: University of Chicago Press.

Jerome, N.W. 1981. The U.S. dietary pattern from an anthropological perspective. *Food Technology* 38(2):37–42.

Lowenberg, M.E., E.N. Todhunter, J.R. Savage, and J.L. Lubawski, 1979. *Food and people* (3rd ed.). New York: John Wiley and Sons.

Tannahill, R. 1973. *Food in history*. New York: Stein and Day.

Figure 4.1
Columbus Lands in the New World

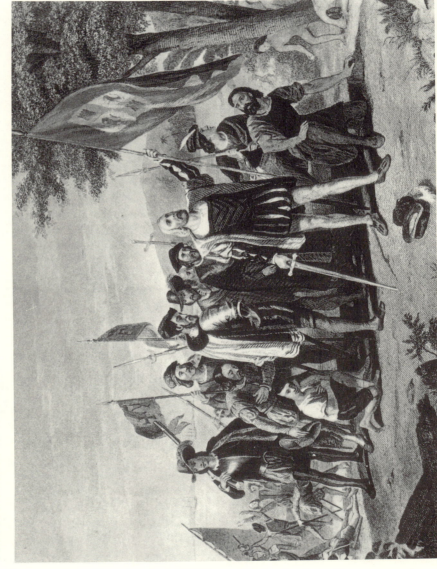

4

Dietary Patterns from Columbian Times Through the American Revolution

EAST MEETS WEST

The Arrival of Columbus

At the time of Columbus's landfall in the Bahamas the morning of October 12, 1492, the Age of Exploration was in full swing in Europe (Figure 4.1). Earlier, in about 1419, Prince Henry of Portugal had established a maritime training center at Sagre, on his country's Atlantic coast. And his passion for navigation had inspired such explorers as Bartholomeu Dias and Vasco da Gama to sail down the coast of Africa and eventually to India (Elson 1992:19). Later, Christopher Columbus, using information gleaned from Ptolemy's maps, attempted what he hoped would be a shorter route to the Orient by sailing westward (Foote 1991). On August 3, 1492, under the flag of Spain the Italian explorer set out from the port of Palos in three ships, the Niña, the Pinta, and the flagship Santa Maria, with a crew of 90 men. He landed on an island in the Bahamas (which he later named San Salvador), on October 12, 1492. This seminal voyage of discovery turned out to be the first of four journeys to what he never believed was a new world. In fact, he never set foot on North America proper. He died in 1506 in Spain, bitter and forgotten, never dreaming that he had discovered any land of significance. Nor did he realize that, one day, this feat would be described as "probably the greatest single addition to human knowledge ever made by one man" (Van Doren 1991:177).

Columbus believed that he had landed on an island of the (East) Indies, near Japan or China. He also believed that the gentle Arawak people, who offered Columbus and his crew ("men from heaven") all they had, were Indians. Although people knew within 30 years that he was wrong, the names have persisted. The native inhabitants of America still are called "Indians," and the island he first reached is recognized as one of the West Indies.

Columbus's Motives for Exploration

Columbus's lifetime (1451–1506) encompassed the end of the Middle Ages, the dawn of Western science, and the birth of modern man. But life still was strikingly different from the present, and modernity was a long way off. During this period, Western Europe was experiencing times of terror, war, pestilence, famine, slavery, and religious persecution (Foote 1991). Its people yearned for a better life.

In addition to the desire for spices, exotic goods, riches, and the possession of new land shared by other explorers of his day, Columbus was driven by religious motives. Although the Crusades had been over since 1270, Columbus hoped to launch, at long last, a final, successful assault on Jerusalem and the Turks—this time from the east. Such religious zeal was in keeping with that of Spain during that momentous year of 1492. Fired with desire for both religious and political gain, Spain was burning heretics, conquering the Moors, and giving tens of thousands of Jews the choice between conversion to Catholicism or expulsion (Armstrong 1988). Thus, it is understandable that Columbus now was able to win the financial support of Ferdinand and Isabella, under whose canny leadership "Spain amassed in the name of Christianity the largest empire the world had ever seen" (Horn and Hawkins 1991:36).

The World Columbus Found

When Columbus set foot on that island of the Bahamas, the technology and other advances of the Old World greatly exceeded those of the New. Yet, both worlds had certain characteristics commonly attributed to Third World areas today. Infant mortality in both worlds was high, and life expectancies were both roughly about 35 per thousand (Glick and Schaefer 1991).

The population of North America at that time has been estimated at between 2 and 18 million people (Dobyus 1983; Ubelaker 1988; Ubelaker 1992:17). And the entire, sparsely populated Western Hemisphere probably had only about as many people as Europe (60–70 million) (Glick and Schaefer 1991; Lord and Burke 1991; Thornton 1987; Ubelaker 1992).

Rather than a new world, Colombus actually discovered another old world, one long populated by numerous, diverse people with distinct cultures (Viola 1991:12). In this strange land, he found brown-skinned people whose ancestors had come over from Asia via the Bering Straits at the time the glacier had receded, some 20,000 to 28,000 years previously (Glick and Schaeffer 1991; Müller-Beck 1967).

Subsequent to their arrival on this continent, the ancestors of these people had experienced four successive archeological periods comprising the prehistoric era—the years between 13000 B.C. and A.D. 1500. It encompasses the Paleo-Indian, Archaic, Woodland Indian, and the Mississippian periods (chapters 3 and 10). These periods apply to almost all geographic areas of what is now the United States (Jerome 1981).

When Columbus arrived, the Indians of what would become the United States generally were into the late Mississippian Period, and their intensive agriculture actually was not too different from that of the early Neolithic peoples of the Old World (Figure 4.2). But while their agriculture was advanced, their domestic animals were few and not very impressive. Alfred Crosby (1972:21) has said, "When Columbus arrived, even the most advanced Indians were barely out of the Stone Age, and their armies were swept aside by tiny bands of conquistadors." The Indians could not compete with the Europeans, who had steel versus their stone, cannons and firearms versus their bows and arrows and slings, and horses. Although horses had originated in North America, they had long been extinct and were now frightening to the Indians (35). Later, however, they began to acquire horses, usually the descendants of those which had escaped from their European owners (Figure 4.3).

It has been estimated that the island of Hispaniola, where Columbus ultimately landed in 1492, had a population of about 250,000 Arawak Indians. But within 20 years, diseases and taskmasters had reduced their number to 14,000 (Lord and Burke 1991:35). By 1600, the native peoples had disappeared (Viola 1991:13).

THE COLUMBIAN EXCHANGE

Columbus's second voyage to the Western world is said to have been the one which changed the world (Glick and Schaefer 1991). Commanding 17 ships, Columbus set sail from Cádiz, Spain, September 25, 1493, with 1,200 men (Crosby 1972:67). They stopped at the Canary Islands, and, resuming their journey, crossed the ocean in just 21 days, arriving November 3, 1493, at an island Columbus named Mariagalante after his flagship. Later, he went on to Hispaniola and founded Isabela on its north coast— the first European colony in America (Morison 1989).

Figure 4.2
Florida Indians Planting Beans of Maize

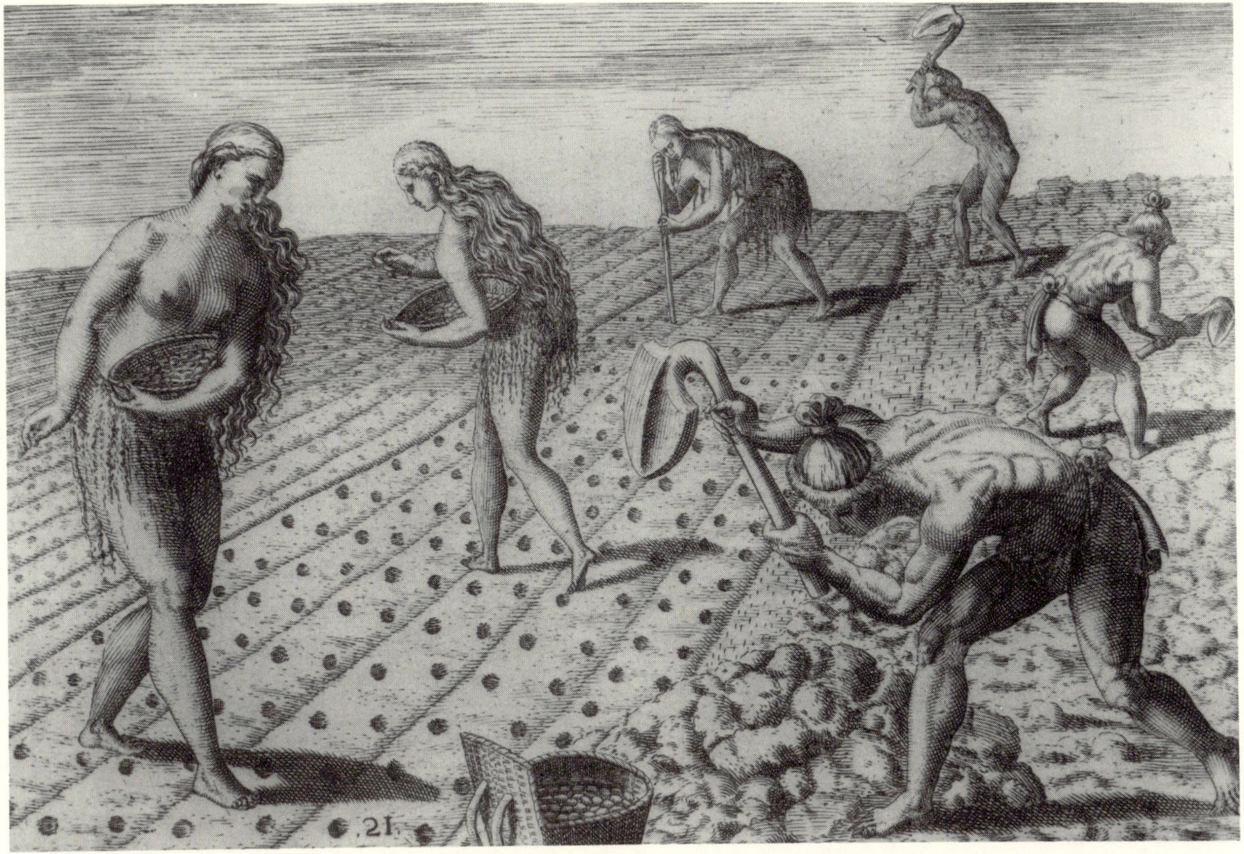

By T. DeBry, 1591. Courtesy of the Library of Congress.

Figure 4.3
Indian Hunting Buffalo

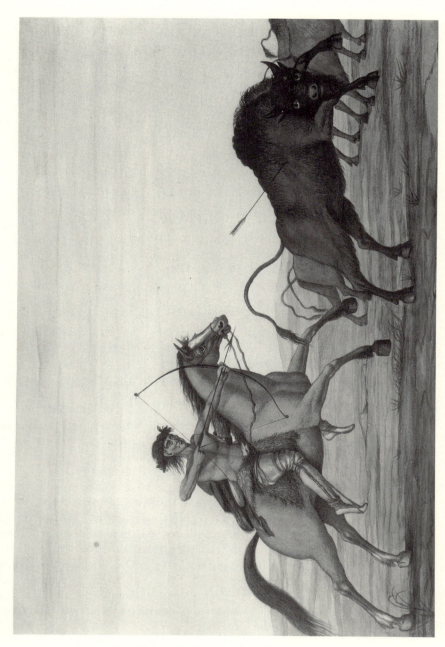

This horse is a descendant of those horses brought by the Europeans. By Peter Rindisbach. State Historical Society of Wisconsin. WHI (X3) 1495.

The first contingent of horses, dogs, pigs, cattle, chickens, sheep, and goats, plus seeds and cuttings, arrived with Columbus on this second voyage in 1493 (Crosby 1972; Glick and Schaefer 1991). This voyage initiated an exchange of flora and fauna between the Eastern and Western hemispheres that has been of unprecedented significance. Europeans brought animals and plants from the Old World, and upon return, carried animals and plants from the New World to the Eastern Hemisphere. "His voyage started the Columbian Exchange, a hemispherical swap of peoples, plants, animals, and diseases that transformed not only the new world that he [Columbus] discovered but also the old one he left" (Glick and Schaefer 1991).

From West to East

Important plant foods. Nikolai Vavilov, the great Russian botanist, in the course of his research on the geographical origin of various cultigens compiled a list of the 640 most important plants cultivated by man. Roughly 500 belonged to the Old World and 100 to the New (Vavilov 1951; Darlington 1963).

Today, over three-fifths of the world's wealth comes from plants unknown to the Eastern Hemisphere before Columbus. While most of these plants are food plants, certain other nonfood plants have had a tremendous economic impact: tobacco, rubber, and certain cottons, indigenous to the New World. Table 4.1 lists the most important plants indigenous to the New World and the Old World, respectively.

Through the Columbian exchanges, people of the Old World became aware of a new staple: maize (corn). Another was manioc (casssava), which was brought by the Portugese from Brazil to Africa in the sixteenth century (Crosby 1972:187). Both of these plant foods were destined to become extremely important staple foods in Africa. Other important New World staples are potatoes and sweet potatoes. Historically, the indigenous staples of the Old World had been rice, wheat, barley, oats, and rye.

In Vavilov's listing of the New World crops he cited fifteen as being the most valuable (1951:39–43) (see Table 4.1). Three of these crops, beans, maize and squash, had constituted the "alimentary trinity" that were supporting the meso-American civilization when the Spanish arrived (Crosby 1972:172). "Collectively, these [fifteen] plants made the most valuable single addition to the food-producing plants of the Old World since the beginnings of agriculture. Of these crops, maize, potatoes, sweet potatoes, beans and manioc (cassava) have been the most abundantly cultivated and eaten in the last 400 years" (170). They are more important to Africa than to any other continent of the Old World, because such a large proportion of its population is dependent on them. Maize and manioc, which arrived in Africa in the sixteenth century, are especially important to Africans

Table 4.1
Most Valuable Crops of the New and Old Worlds

New World[1]	Old World[2]
Maize	Wheat
Beans of many kinds	Rice
Peanuts	Barley
Potato	Oats
Sweet potato	Rye
Manioc (cassava)	Sorghum
Squashes	Millet
Pumpkin	Bananas
Papaya	Cane sugar
Guava	Coffee
Avocado	Eggplant
Pineapple	
Tomato	
Chile pepper	
Cocoa	

[1]N.I. Vavilov, 1951:39–43.
[2]A.W. Crosby, 1972; S.A. Goldblith, 1992.

(185–86). The American crops of primary importance in Europe have been potatoes, followed by beans and maize. Indian plants made a uniquely valuable contribution to the cultigens of the Old World by providing an increased variety of plants from which farmers could produce needed food (175–77).

It is believed that, because America had so few domesticated animals suitable for food, the Indians may have been driven to focus intensively on plants for subsistence. This circumstance thus resulted in the development of some of the most important of all plants (170). In addition, the Indians also gave humanity such nonfood plants as tobacco, rubber, and certain cottons (Vavilov 1951).

From East to West

Important plant foods. The Columbian exchange was a two-way street. Plant cultigens from the Old World that have been of great socioeconomic importance to the Western Hemisphere are listed in Table 4.1. Of these, rice, wheat, barley, oats, and rye had been staples in the Old World. Other foods, perhaps more exotic, that have come from the Eastern Hemisphere include bananas, cane sugar, coffee, and eggplant. The latter is one of the few plants of the nightshade family that did not originate in the Americas (Goldblith 1992:74). Today, the largest crops, worldwide, are wheat, rice, maize, potatoes, and barley, in that order (see Table 2.1).

By 1600, all the most important food plants of the Old World were being grown in America. This situation is due in large part to the European colonists' desire for a dependable supply of their native, familiar European food. Without this successful transference of European agriculture to the Western Hemisphere, the number of Europeans willing to emigrate to America would have been far smaller (Crosby 1972:106–7).

Unquestionably, the immigrant flora vastly enriched the food-producing potential of America. For example, rice enabled Americans to make better use of swampy soils, where the New World staples—maize and manioc—do not grow well. In another instance, Americans living in mountainous areas benefited from wheat, barley, and European broadbeans, which grow at altitudes higher than maize (106).

Influx of new animals. Important though plants from the Old World were, the animals brought by Columbus and his followers were even more valuable. Thanks to the efforts of the Spanish conquistadors, all of the leading domesticated species (including horses and cattle) had arrived by 1500. These domesticated animals now supplied the colonists with meat in amounts greater than perhaps any other non-nomadic people in the world. Pigs did especially well, and their descendants proliferate today (Glick and Schaefer 1991). Livestock, fortunately, were able to convert grass into foods for humans: meat, milk, and cheese. Thus, the coming of European animals created a dramatic increase in the quantity of animal protein available for human consumption in America (Crosby 1972:108).

The Columbian exchange made possible a dietary variety and a nutritional status never before dreamed of. Unquestionably, there is a connection between Columbus's voyages and the population explosion of the past 300 years (165–66; Goldblith 1992: 85).

THE COLONIAL PERIOD (1500–1783)

Although most of the colonists were English, the North America American continent also attracted thousands of Europeans of Dutch, French, German, Scotch-Irish, Scottish, Spanish, and Swedish origins. The Spanish and French were interested mainly in furs, gold, and other riches. They were interested also in converting the Indians to Roman Catholicism. A primary motive for most of the colonists was that of economic opportunity: finding work, farmland, and a place to settle. Some settlers came to America to find freedom of worship because they had been persecuted in their homelands for their religious beliefs. They included the Pilgrims, Quakers, some Roman Catholics, Huguenots, and Jews. Most of the English colonists wanted to set up permanent homes and engage in agriculture.

As settlers adjusted to their new homes, the Indians were helpful in many ways, particularly with respect to obtaining an adequate food supply and teaching the colonists their methods of intensive agriculture. However, there also was much hostility and fighting, as the Indians became aware that the Europeans were taking over land which they perceived as their own. The colonists eventually drove the Indians west and took over the land. They produced plenty of food and other items on their farms and plantations. The colonists carried on a thriving trade with England and other countries and built homes, villages, and cities. They also established churches, schools, and local governments.

By the end of the Colonial Period, the living conditions of most colonists were equal to those of prosperous people in Europe's wealthiest nations. Moreover, they had more freedom to govern themselves than did any other people of that period.

Spanish Colonizers

The Spanish became the first colonizers in America when Columbus brought 1,500 settlers to the island of Hispaniola on his second voyage in 1493. He brought cuttings of sugar cane to the Western Hemisphere on this voyage and planted them in Santo Domingo, now the capital of the Dominican Republic. He also brought the sweet orange. Hispaniola became a base for further Spanish expansion into Florida, Mexico, and Peru. The Spanish also explored areas of Texas, New Mexico, and Arizona. St. Augustine, in Florida, was established in 1565, the oldest permanent European settlement in the country. The orange was growing there as early as 1579. These Spanish colonizers found chocolate, which the Aztecs had in Mexico, and later introduced it to North America and Europe.

English Colonizers

Although the English arrived relatively late in America, they were the first Europeans to settle in large numbers (Martin 1989a:4, 786). Between 1607 and 1733, the English established 13 permanent colonies on the Atlantic coast of North America (Table 4.2). These early settlements developed mainly through business projects managed by English businessmen or companies who had obtained permits from the king to colonize lands in the New World. The primary objectives of these colonizers were to make money and to expand English trade and industry. Promoting America as a land of opportunity, they persuaded many Europeans to come to the colonies. Often, these merchants provided the immigrants with transportation, land, and tools (787).

The English colonies. The colonies are grouped generally according to location: (1) the Northern or New England colonies, (2) the Middle colonies, and (3) the Southern colonies.

The Northern colonies were Connecticut, Massachusetts, New Hampshire, and Rhode Island. Most New Englanders lived in villages and had

Table 4.2
The English Colonies of the Atlantic Coast

Colony	First Permanent Settlement
Virginia	1607
Massachusetts	1620
New Hampshire	1623
New York	1624
Connecticut	1633
Maryland	1634
Rhode Island	1636
Delaware	1638
Pennsylvania	1643
North Carolina	1650
New Jersey	1660
South Carolina	1670
Georgia	1733

small farms. The climate was cool and the soil rocky. However, New England colonies had plenty of fine timber and some of the best fishing waters in the world.

The Middle colonies were Delaware, New Jersey, New York, and Pennsylvania. The soil and climate in this area were suitable for large farms, where wheat and other grains were grown.

The Southern colonies were Georgia, Maryland, North Carolina, South Carolina, and Virginia. The warm climate and rich soil of the South were ideal for growing tobacco and rice, often on large plantations.

History and Eating Patterns of Selected Colonies

Virginia. Jamestown was the first permanent English colony in America. In 1607, nine ships with 800 passengers and crew set sail from England for Virginia. They brought with them cheese, cured fish and meat, oatmeal, bread and biscuits, beans and onions, dried fruits, seasonings, and butter (which probably spoiled on the way). Also, they brought barrels of beer, cider, and water and seeds for future planting. Six hundred fifty immigrants actually reached what now is called Jamestown Island. The Indians brought the colonists gifts of corn and taught them where fish could be caught and what wild game was edible. An Indian named Squanto is reputed to have been especially helpful to the Pilgrims in this regard. However, food still was inadequate. So many settlers died during the winter of 1609–10 that it became known as the "starving times." By 1617, additional immigration had increased the population to 4,000(Lowenberg, Todhunter, Wilson, Feeney, and Savage 1968:66). In spite of hardships, Jamestown survived, and a sister settlement developed at Williamsburg.

Planters and their families eventually replaced the original explorers and traders who had settled in Virginia. Tobacco lured new colonists because there was a good market in England for Virginia tobacco. Almost everyone in Virginia became involved in tobacco farming. But the methods used in growing tobacco so seriously depleted the soil that this crop could not be grown on a given plot more than three years. Unfortunately, instead of restoring old land, the colonists preferred to clear new land. So they (and their farms) moved westward.

In the spring of the year, the colonists found that the first and most important task was to plant a garden and a field of corn. Since the Indians' squash and pumpkins were easy to grow, they were commonly planted in the gardens. Corn was the staple grain of both the colony and the frontier. It was a food plant thus far unknown to Europeans and Asians, whose staples historically had been primarily wheat, rice, and barley. The Indians taught the settlers how to grind their corn by using a mortar and pestle. The mortar was a hole formed in a stump, and the pestle was a log. From the Indians, the colonists learned that cracked corn could be made into hominy and many other dishes.

The first hogs in the colony were brought in 1652. They were well adapted to both the colonies and the frontier, since they could survive on kitchen waste and forest acorns, from oak trees. Later, they were allowed to roam widely and to eat the peanuts grown by the planters. The nearer the frontier, the more important game became. Beef and game were dried according to the traditional methods of the Indians (Lowenberg et al.:67).

African slaves. Increased trade in Virginia spurred increased production and the need for a larger labor force. But by the 1600s Indian slavery essentially had been abolished. Instead, the colonists began to use Africans and indentured white servants to care for the labor-intensive tobacco and cotton crops. The first Africans were brought to Virginia in 1619 by a Dutch ship. Later, they were introduced into other colonies (Jernegan 1959: 87). The sizable addition of Africans to the population of the South had a significant impact on its economic and social structure.

New York. The Dutch established the fur trading post of New Amsterdam on Manhattan Island in 1613. Later, the Dutch East India Company offered tracts of land along the Hudson River to any ship's officer who would transport fifty settlers to the new colony at his own expense. In March 1623, thirteen families of Walloons from southern and southeastern Belgium and France arrived in New Amsterdam. During the first year, they were able to survive through the help of the Indians, who brought them gifts of corn and provided guidance in procuring game and seafood from the environment. In April of the following year, an expedition of three ships brought additional settlers with needed agricultural and dairy equipment. This expedition also carried 100 head of livestock, horses, hogs, and sheep. The Dutch were well organized, and both the voyage and subsequent settlements of the colonizers were well managed. The fertile soil lent itself to the raising of grain, tobacco, fruit, and a wide variety of vegetables, including the native beans, pumpkin, and squash.

Massachusetts. The Pilgrims landed at Plymouth in November 1620 and developed the second permanent English settlement in America. This group was in search of religious freedom. It has been said that a shortage of beer and its adverse effects on the sailors' morale had much to do with the diverting of the Mayflower from its original destination, at the Virginia colony, further south. Much of their food had spoiled, so they had little left. And the shelter they were able to find for the winter was poor. Like the settlers at Jamestown, the Pilgrims suffered from both disease and famine during their first winter. Only about half of the original 99 settlers survived.

Fortunately, the Pilgrims soon developed good relations with the local Indians, who were particularly helpful in teaching them how to raise corn and the locations of the best fishing areas. The Indians gave the colonists corn, taught them how to raise beans with the corn and then to store the ears in ventilated cribs and grind the corn. By this time, corn, sweet potatoes, pumpkins, and squash had been raised by the North American Indians for generations. Root crops were introduced by the settlers themselves. Fish were abundant in the Atlantic and the nearby rivers. Meals were mainly the one-pot type. One year later, the Plymouth colony celebrated a day of Thanksgiving, with a feast of corn bread, cranberries, wild turkey, and pumpkin baked in maple syrup (Lowenberg et al. 1968:68–69). (The wild turkey during this period ranged from Mexico to northern New England. Originally hunted by the Aztecs in Mexico, they had found their way to Europe by 1530. Seafaring Turks had picked them up and then took them to England. Hence, the birds became known as "turkeys"). Venison became less plentiful as the colony grew, because of overhunting.

After English colonists had settled Jamestown and Plymouth, large areas of the Atlantic seacoast were colonized. The later colonists suffered hardships, but in general nowhere as severe as those experienced at Jamestown and Plymouth (Martin 1989a:4,790).

Delaware. The Swedes developed the first settlements along the Delaware River in 1638. The early settlers were fur traders. But, in 1655, after years of friction with the Dutch fur traders of New York, the Swedes turned their attention to fruit and tobacco raising and small farming. Blessed with fertile soil, the Swedes became successful in growing fruit and gardens of beans, peas, and cabbage. In addition to the rye of their native land, they raised barley, corn, wheat in Delaware, as well as cows, goats, and sheep. They enjoyed beer, produced from their own corn; excellent native wine, cow's and goat's milk, and shellfish.

New Jersey. In 1664, about 230 families of Quakers arrived from England, Ireland, and Scotland, destined for farmlands then available on liberal terms. Part of New Jersey was originally intended as a retreat for Quakers intent upon a peaceful life in a new country. They were well-to-do, practical, industrious, and thrifty people, who lived a sober, modest life. But like all of the American colonists, they were faced with the need to find food and shelter upon their arrival. The Indians supplied them with their first corn. Fish were plentiful. But they did not pursue game, since the Quakers were not hunters. Native cranberries and blueberries soon became important crops, for which New Jersey still is well known. Under the husbandry of the Quakers the fertile soil produced many good crops of grain, vegetables, and fruit. New Jersey came to be known as the Garden State. Food was good and abundant.

Pennsylvania. The Germans came to America during the seventeenth century and the early and mid-eighteenth century. Some of the earliest arrivals settled in New York. Later, welcomed by the Quaker William Penn, they moved west to land in southeast Pennsylvania. These Germans, or Pennsylvania Dutch (from "Deutch," meaning German), were born farmers, committed to hard work. They raised all their own food, buying only salt and spices. Soup, bread, and vegetables were the first foods of the early pioneers. Later, they were able to add milk, wild game, fowl, wild berries, and preserves to their diet. Tea was brewed from herbs; coffee was made from burnt rye or wheat, and their butter was cottage cheese. In time, the daily fare of the established Pennsylvania Dutch household reflected choices from an impressive variety of foods. They included bread, milk, cornmeal, potato and noodle soup, pork with sauerkraut or dumplings, sausage, liverwurst, bread and apple fritters, pancakes, sausage meat, molasses, syrup, farm jelly, applesauce, cottage cheese, salads, and a wide choice of pie and cake (Lowenberg et al. 1968:70–71).

Colonial Food Habits: An Overview

Aid from the Indians. When Columbus and the early white settlers arrived, the Eastern Atlantic and Florida Indians were advanced horticulturists. They also were adept at food gathering: hunting, fishing, and collecting. The early settlers owe much to the Indians, who taught them where and how to fish, hunt, and collect food, in addition to sharing with them their agricultural expertise. They taught the colonists much about what crops to raise and how to raise them. They taught the Pilgrims to plant corn in a hill and then to form a row of hills. They demonstrated how to fertilize each hill with a dead fish. They also taught them to plant beans, peanuts, and vine crops between the rows of corn. This practice enabled the plants to benefit from a symbiotic relationship: the corn provided shade and protection for the low-growing plants, while the nitrogen-fixing legumes provided the corn with much-needed nitrogen. Some of the

Indians had learned to make corn cribs from tree limbs, for drying and storing corn.

Such advice was especially valuable to the colonists, who were mainly ex-tradespeople and craftsmen. Except for the Germans, who were true farmers, the colonists knew little about hunting, fishing, and agriculture, particularly in the New World.

History gives us glimpses of Indian women teaching their cooking skills to the early white female settlers cooking with whom they lived side by side (Jones 1990:8). From them the newcomers learned the many ways of preparing corn and beans (succotash, corn pone and other more complicated corn breads, soups, and stews) and the principles of outdoor cooking. The white women settlers adopted some of these dishes carte blanche; they integrated others and adapted them into their own recipes. The Indians' custom of the one-dish meal and their practice of cooking food outdoors over an open fire, using spits, were already familiar to them from Britain (Figure 4.4.). So they adopted these methods without hesitation, especially in view of their scanty utensils and fuel sources.

In balance, despite fighting and skirmishes between Indians and colonists during the Colonial years, the Indian played an essential role in enabling the colonists to adapt successfully to the New World. Without their aid, the colonists would not have obtained an adequate food supply.

Colonial food supply. After the difficult early years of food scarcity and adjustment to a new land, food became generally plentiful. In fact, the colonists kept themselves better supplied with food than any other people in the world. James Martin (1989a:796–97) has provided this description of colonial food habits:

On their farms, they raised grain, cattle, hogs, sheep, chickens, fruits, and vegetables. In the fields and woodlands, they hunted deer, pigeons, squirrels, wild turkeys, and other game. From the river and ocean waters, they took clams, oysters, lobsters, and many kinds of fish.

Corn was a basic food in almost every household. The people ate it in many forms, most commonly as corn bread. A woman mixed corn meal with water or milk, salt, and lard, and shaped it into buns. Then she baked or fried the buns on a hoe or on a griddle, or placed them in the ashes of the fireplace. Corn bread had different names in various parts of colonial America—ash-cake, hoecake, johny-cake, or corn pone. Cooks also made corn hominy. Sometimes they roasted ears of corn in the husks.

Rye or wheat bread was made with yeast. In many homes, the women baked these breads in a small oven that was built into the fireplace or outside the house, against the hot chimney. They also baked bread in an iron bake kettle, which had a tight-fitting lid. The kettle stood on a bed of hot coals, with embers piled around it and on top of the lid.

Meat or game was usually cooked with vegetables into a stew. Women made the stew in a large iron pot that hung over the fire on a pothook, fastened to a crane

Figure 4.4
"The Broyling of Their Fish over the Flame of Fier"

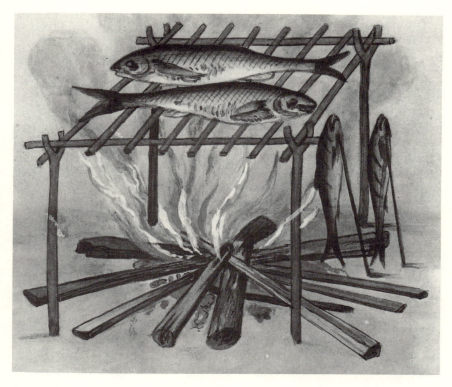

By John White (1585–1587). John White was a member of an expedition sent by Sir Walter Raleigh in 1585 to the new settlement at Roanoke. Raleigh had specifically instructed White to sketch local life around the area. Courtesy of the Library of Congress.

or a chimney bar. The iron pot had short legs and sometimes was placed on a bed of coals. Whole fowl or large cuts of meat were often roasted on sharp-pointed rods called spits. Handles on the spits allowed the meat to be turned above the fire.

Food preparation and preservation. Food usually was prepared by boiling, roasting, steaming, or baking. Drying, salting, pickling, and cooling were the major methods used in preservation. The diet varied markedly by season and climate. Since the colonists did not yet have methods of canning or refrigeration, storing food for the winter was a problem. Some meat (especially pork) could be successfully salted or smoked, while certain vegetables were dried or pickled. Root vegetables and certain fruits (e.g., apples) were kept in cool, dry cellars. Bread and meat often were the standbys during winter (Martin 1989a:4,797). "The diet at times, particularly in

Figure 4.5
Colonial Kitchen, Williamsburg, Virginia

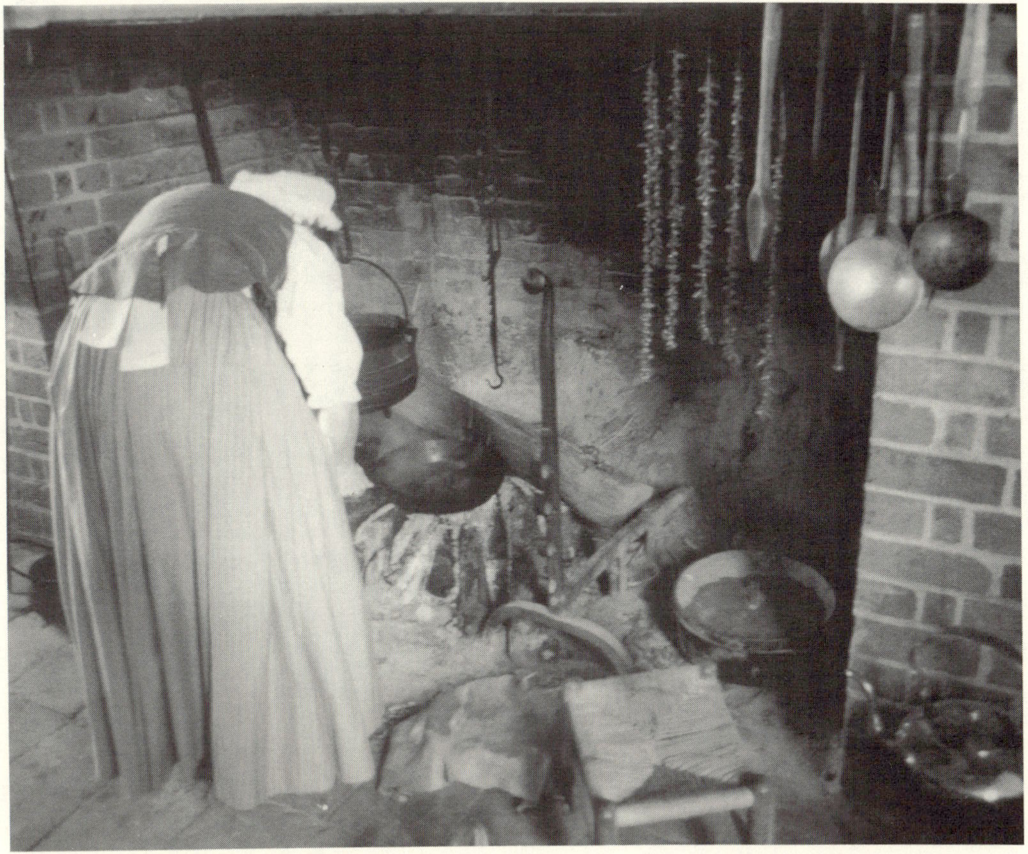

Photographed by Nancy Sell

winter, must have had little variety, but there seems to have been relatively little actual want" (Van Syckle 1945a:19,508).

Beverages. The colonists drank large amounts of beer, cider, rum, or wine with all their meals, rather than water. They believed, as did most Europeans of the day, that their water was unsafe to drink. The most popular alcoholic beverage of the colonists was Madeira wine, imported from the Portuguese island of the same name. By the 1700s, tea, coffee, and hot chocolate were popular beverages (Martin 1989a:4,797–798).

Food and social status. During colonial times, certain dietary variations related to social status. Three criteria served to distinguish the diets of the well-to-do from those less affluent in Colonial New England: type and color of bread, quality and source of animal protein, and frequency of consuming butter (Jerome 1981:39). "The diet of the well-to-do included fresh meat, white bread and butter, while that of those less well-to-do included salted meat, fish, baked beans, Indian-meal bread, and rye (dark) bread" (Van Syckle 1945a:21,509).

The Colonial dietary pattern. The food production system that emerged during the Colonial period resulted from the merging of two different agricultural traditions—the Indian and European. Food was central to the European's adjustment in the new land. And the colonists' success in obtaining an abundant and varied diet was made possible by utilizing various techniques, representing a blend of Indian and European technologies, in producing, processing, and preparing foods. The colonial period has been credited with providing the basic structure of a dominant American dietary pattern, which still persists. This pattern consists of animal meat as the central entree, augmented by fruits, vegetables, grain products, dairy products, legumes, sweetmeats, sugar, and alcohol (Jerome 1981:39).

THE AMERICAN REVOLUTION (1775–1783)

The Revolutionary War led to the birth of a new, independent nation: the United States of America. Before its onset, tension had been building for more than 10 years between Great Britain and the American Colonies. Beginning in the mid-1760s, the British government passed a series of laws to increase its control over the colonies. By this time, the colonists had become accustomed to a large degree of self-government and strongly resisted the new laws. They were especially opposed to the tax laws. In 1775, Britain's Parliament declared Massachusetts, the site of much protest, to be in rebellion. The British government ordered its troops to take swift action against the rebels. War broke out soon after that. On July 4, 1776, the Second Continental Congress adopted the Declaration of Independence, whereby the Colonies broke ties with the mother country, and formed the United States. On September 3, 1783, Britain signed the Treaty of Paris, by which it recognized the independence of the United States (and whereby the Colonies became an independent nation). This treaty also established the new nation's borders. The United States now extended west to the Mississippi River, north to Canada, east to the Atlantic Ocean, and south to Florida. Britain gave Florida to Spain (Martin 1989b:16,274–91).

FOR FURTHER READING

Crosby, A.W. 1972. *The Columbian exchange.* Westport, CT: Greenwood Press.

Elson, J. 1992. The millennium of discovery. *Time*, Fall 1992, 16–26.

Foote, T. 1991. Where Columbus was coming from. *Smithsonian* 22 (9):28–41.

Goldblith, S.A. 1992. The legacy of Columbus, with particular reference to foods. *Food Technology* 46(10):62–85.

Lowenberg, M.E., E.N. Todhunter, E.D. Wilson, M.C. Feeney, and J.R. Savage. 1968. *Food and people.* New York: John Wiley and Sons.

Martin, J.K. 1989a. Colonial life in America. *World Book Encyclopedia* 4:786–813. Chicago: World Book.

Van Syckle, C. 1945a. Some pictures of food consumption in the United States: Part I, 1630–1860. *Journal of the Am. Diet. Assoc.* 19:508–512.

Vavilov, N.I. 1951. *The origin, variation, immunity and breeding of cultivated plants.* New York: Ronald Press Company.

Verano, J.W., and D.H. Ubelaker (eds.). 1992. *Disease and Demography in the Americas.* Washington: Smithsonian Institution Press.

Viola, H.J., and C. Margolis. 1991. *Seeds of change.* Washington: Smithsonian Institution Press.

5

American Food Habits: The New Republic Through the Nineteenth Century

THE UNITED STATES: A NEW INDEPENDENT REPUBLIC (1783–1850)

During the early years of the republic, the United States still was essentially rural. In 1800, approximately 95 percent of the population lived on small farms.

Important Developments

Agricultural change. By the nineteenth century, major developments were beginning to take place in the agricultural economy. The Industrial Revolution, which began in Britain in the 1700s, was moving to America. By 1830, industrialization was affecting not only urban areas and its factories. It also was changing the face of agriculture. Norge Jerome (1981:40) has noted that the social, economic, intellectual, and political vitality that followed the Revolutionary War stimulated technological advancements in farm equipment and in plant and animal agriculture. The formation of land and agricultural societies led to a greater organization of agriculture. There was a growing conviction that food scarcity was no longer inevitable. According to Jerome, these developments did not have an immediate impact on the diet, which still did not differ greatly from colonial eating patterns. But, since 1800, land-hungry European immigrants had been pouring into

**Figure 5.1
Slave Sitting by a Fireplace**

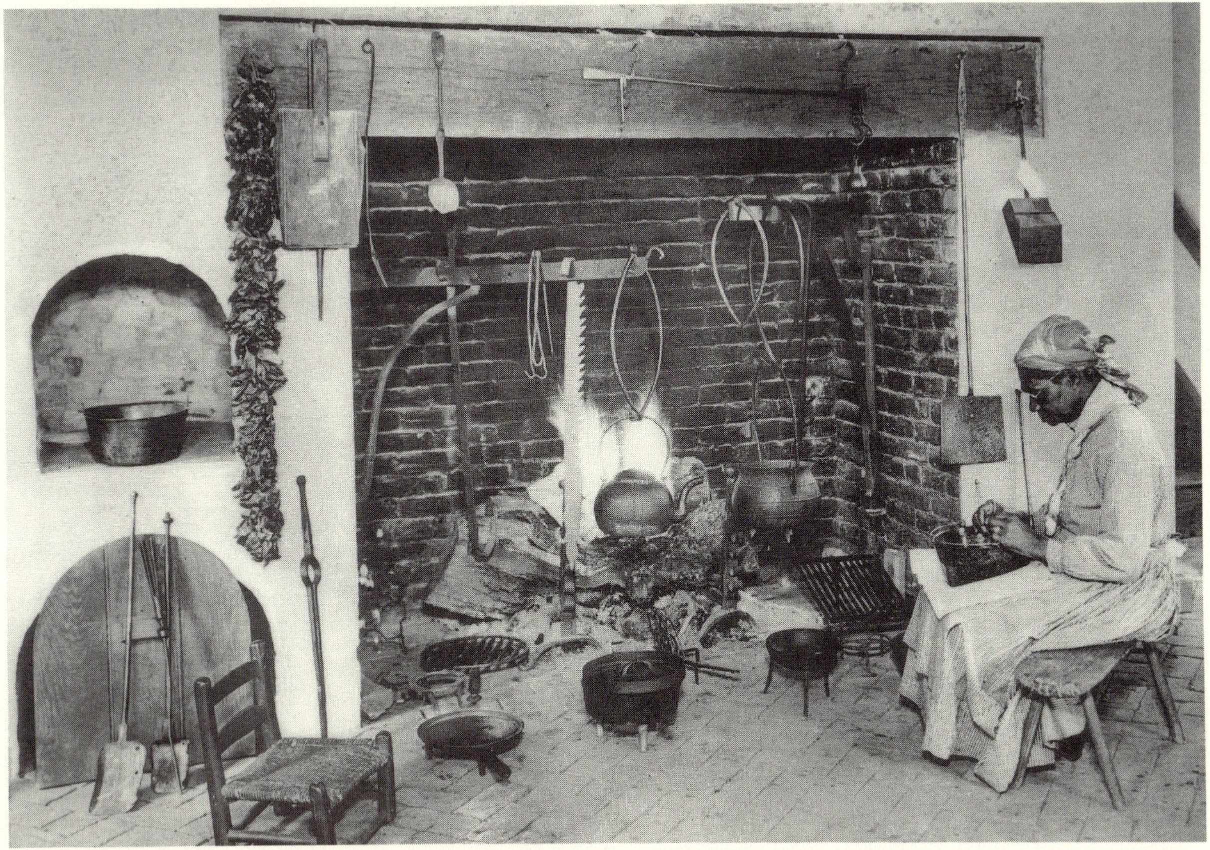

America, which promised freedom and land for the asking. The ensuing population growth along with the changing social environment and organization later exerted a direct influence on the food system and dietary patterns (40).

Technological advances. Numerous important inventions during this period had a positive effect on agriculture and the food system. Jethro Wood, a New York farmer, invented the iron moldboard bottom plow in 1819. John Deere, an Illinois blacksmith, produced the first steel plow in 1837. Cyrus McCormick invented the reaper in 1832. Later, a binder and the J. J. Case threshing machine were developed. Modern mechanized farming followed.

Meanwhile, the invention of the cooking range by Massachusetts-born Benjamin Thompson during the late eighteenth century, was beginning to affect food preparation in the home. By 1840 or 1850, old fireplaces were falling into disuse for cooking, replaced by wood- and coal-burning ranges. Later, cooking was made even easier, when the latter gave way to ranges run by gas or electricity (Lowenberg et al. 1979:79). Ice was used increasingly for preserving food, following the invention of an ice-cooled refrigerator by Thomas Moore, a Maryland farmer, in 1803 (Cummings 1970: 36–37) (Figure 5.2). John Dutton patented a process for making artificial ice in 1846 (Lowenberg et al. 1979:79).

Indians. During the early and mid-1800s, advancing white settlers claimed more and more Indian lands. To free more land for settlement, Congress passed the Indian Removal Act in 1830. This act allowed the president to move the eastern Indian tribes to land west of the Mississippi River. This region, which the U.S. government set aside for the residence of Indians between 1830 and 1906, was designated as Indian territory. It was thinly settled and considered to be of little value. The U.S. government moved more than 70,000 Indians across the Mississippi to newly established reservations. Thousands of Indians died on the journey westward. The trip made by the five Cherokee tribes became known as the Trail of Tears.

Eating Patterns of the Period

The diet pattern of this period was very similar to that of the preceding colonial period (Jerome 1981:39–40). Because of the narrow range of foods consumed by most British Americans before the mid-nineteenth century, a number of modern writers have viewed the diet of this period as monotonous, as well as bland and heavy (e.g., Martin 1942:54–55 and Volney 1804:323). Constantin Volney, a French traveler, criticized the food of many early nineteenth-century Americans as being monotonous and poorly prepared. Herbs and spices were used sparsely. Frying was a common

Figure 5.2
Message for the Iceman

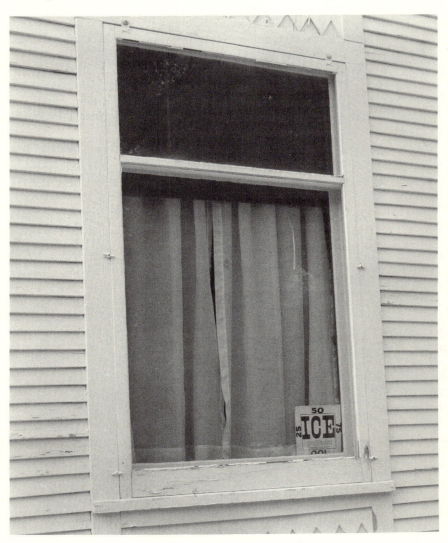

Photographed by Tom McIntosh

method of preparing food, and the resultant grease often was reserved for the making of sauces and gravies.

Samuel Eliot Morison (1965:473) has this to say about the diet during the early half of the nineteenth century: "American cooking at this period

Table 5.1
Waves of Immigration in the United States

Wave	Period	Number of Immigrants	Major Countries of Origin
First	1830–1860	4,900,000	Germany, Great Britain, Ireland
Second	1860–1890	10,000,000	Germany, Great Britain, Ireland, Scandinavia
Third	1890–1930	22,000,000	Greece, Austria-Hungary, Italy, Poland, Portugal, Russia, Spain

Source: M. Rischin, 1989.

was generally bad, and the diet worse." According to Waverly Root and Richard de Rochement (1976:132), foreign observers of the American diet during this period granted that if the food was not good, it was at least abundant.

During this period, the diet varied according to geographic region, season, and socioeconomic level. Rural and urban diets differed, as did racial and ethnic diets of this period (Van Syckle 1945a). Between 1830 and 1860, almost 5 million immigrants had arrived (Table 5.1), who brought in new eating habits. The population was growing. Regional foods continued to develop as the population dispersed. Despite these diversities, certain generalizations can be made.

Rural population. The country was still overwhelmingly rural. Most people lived on small farms and produced their own food, except for sugar, salt, and spices which they obtained from the country general store. The diet remained very similar to that of the previous colonial period.

The mainstay of the American diet was the indigenous corn and potatoes, along with pork, bread, and butter. These foods served as staples in the well-settled sections, as well as on the frontier.

Corn was the main cereal grain since wheat crops were often damaged by the "blast," a smut that damaged the crop in much of New England during this time. Cornmeal was used in many ways, as during colonial times (see chapter 4).

In the Midwest during the 1830s, a Mrs. Trollope found that corn was eaten in many forms—in hominy, as well as in a dozen different cakes—all of them bad, she said (Trollope 1832b:130–31). However, she acknowledged that a bread utilizing one part meal to two parts flour yielded by far the best bread she had ever tasted. The pioneers found that corn was easy to grow on the frontier, even before land had been completely cleared, since corn could be planted, and grew well, between the stumps remaining from felled trees. In the South, corn was considered more valuable than gold, since it was eaten by everything, "from slave to chick" (Martineau 1837: 43–44).

In the North, white or Irish potatoes were eaten. In the South, the white potato was not grown, because it matured and had to be dug relatively early in the season, when it was too hot for successful storage in the warm southern climate. Instead, the sweet potato, which did not mature until autumn, constituted the staple starch. It was then harvested, and stored, fried, roasted, candied, or made into custard.

Richard Cummings has stated that "land was cheap and meat abundant in the America of 1789" (1970:15). Pork was the favorite meat throughout the United States during this time, not only in the well-settled areas of New England and the South, but also on the frontier. There were some compelling reasons for its popularity. Pigs were easy for the settlers to keep, either by feeding them from their usually abundant supplies of corn, or allowing them to roam free, as did the southern mountaineers. With the latter management style, the pigs picked up their own living from acorns and other fodder in forested areas, in all seasons, and required no attention at all (Kephart 1929:16). The pig yielded a quick return, maturing quickly. Pork was valued not only for its excellent taste, but for its good keeping qualities. Whereas keeping most meats was a problem in this prerefrigeration era, pork was unique because it lent itself so well to such preservation processes as smoking and salting. In fact, its flavor actually improved as a result of these treatments.

In general, beef was much less used than pork, in part because it was more expensive. However, among prosperous New Englanders, the use of the two meats appears to have been about equal (Goodrich 1850:80). Mutton was well liked, but because of its poor keeping qualities was infrequently available.

Except for occasional game, fresh meats were generally available only at slaughtering time. Fresh meat was so likely to be tainted that it is easy to understand why a reliable store of preserved pork, however salty, was much preferred.

Meat consumption (mainly pork) was high. It has been estimated that per capita meat consumption during the 1830–39 decade was 178 pounds annually (48 pounds more than was eaten in 1930), or about 0.5 pound daily (Cummings 1970:15).

The year-round availability of milk was hindered in New England by the use of open pasturage during the early nineteenth century. Using this practice, which had been traditional in England, milk became scarce when grass became winter killed. Milk intake generally was inadequate, by current nutrition standards.

When milk was available, that not used immediately often was converted to butter and cheese in the homes, using churns and cheese presses. Compared to milk, cheese and butter could be kept for long periods. In this way, the use of milk could be maximized. However, rancidity was a frequent problem, especially in dairy products. Milk was a great rarity in the South because of the difficulty of keeping it fresh in hot weather (Martineau 1837:44, 49).

In the well-settled areas, fresh vegetables sometimes were served in season. However, they were rather casually and sparingly used, usually as a side dish or "sass," according to British tradition. Moreover, since leafy vegetables would keep only a short time, most of the vegetables consumed were those which could be stored in bins or preserved by drying (Lutes 1936:211–12). Examples were turnips, pumpkins, and beans. In the south, chickpeas were widely eaten.

Farmers had little fresh fruit, especially in winter. Wild berries were available in spring and summer. Unfortunately, orchard fruits tended to be raised specifically for the making of cider and brandy. Most fruits were so perishable that they had to be preserved pound for pound with sugar (a costly process) or dried. The exception was apples. Since they could be stored for several months, they were the most common fruit in winter. However, on the frontier, orchard fruit did not become available for some years because of the time it takes for fruit trees to mature. In 1833, it was noted that even on the seaboard, few farmers had many fruit trees (Cummings 1970:21).

Some farmers on the coast drank tea or coffee and bought brown sugar or molasses (a by-product of the sugar industry) for sweetening. On the frontier, before coffee became available, coffeelike beverages were made from roasted wheat or other grains.

Along the seacoast, breweries and cider mills provided beer and cider. However, in the back country, the making of these beverages was prevented by the lack of both apples and facilities for keeping malt liquor. Instead, corn (fermented and distilled into liquor) provided whiskey, which became a much-used drink among the pioneers (1970:17). According to Thomas Ashe (1808:241), Kentuckians drank ardent spirits, or strong distilled liquors, from morning until night.

As single cash croppers, the tobacco farmers of Virginia invested little time, energy, or land in the raising of food crops. As a result, both men and animals were "illy fed," according to Thomas Jefferson (Ford 1894: 271).

Morison (1965:503) has noted (with respect to the 1820–50 period) that "although the gentry gave the tone to Southern white society, there were relatively few of them, probably not more than 15,000 families." According to this historian, the typical southerner was a farmer who, with perhaps a half dozen slaves, cultivated a cash crop and also produced a large part of his own food. In addition, there were several hundred thousand southern families who owned no slaves. Hence, there were wide variations in the diets among the various socioeconomic classes. The wealthy plantation owner's diet was varied and abundant, although fashion and convenience called for slave women to serve as wet nurses for the babies of well-to-do mothers. Small slave owners and non-slave-holding yeomen lived in double log cabins or bare framehouses without conveniences, on a diet largely of "hog 'n' hominy." This sort of diet often produced pellagra, because of its lack of niacin (or tryptophan, its precursor). This deficiency disease later assumed proportions large enough to become a serious public health problem by the turn of the century.

The occurrence of pellagra also was exacerbated by lack of milk, which is a good source of tryptophan, from which the body can synthesize the vitamin niacin. Milk, like other perishable foods, was scarce in the South because it did not keep well in warm weather (Schafer 1936:48).

Slaves had a still different diet. Often, it was more nutritious than that of the poor white farmer. House servants tended to eat from the food prepared in the master's kitchen, while field slaves lived and prepared meals in their own cabins. The latter were especially likely to have their own small garden plots. They ate vegetables from these gardens, plus discarded vegetable and meat parts from the plantation owner's kitchen. Moreover, they used the pot liquor (rich in vitamins and minerals) left over from the cooking of meat scraps and vegetables to make gravies. The slaves learned to make adroit use of spices to add zest to these humble foodstuffs. Many of the dishes were so tasty that they began to be served by the cooks in the masters' dining rooms as well. In our own time, these dishes have come to be called soul food (see chapter 9). These "leavings" often provided enough niacin to protect the slaves from developing pellagra (chapter 6) and also enough other vitamins and minerals to protect them against many other nutritional deficiencies common during this era.

Urban population. The diets of city dwellers were even lower in milk, fresh fruits, and vegetables than rural diets. Methods of supplying perishable foods to the markets were primitive at the beginning of the nineteenth century. Until railroad service arrived, supplies of fruits and vegetables in Boston, New York, and other cities were scarce in the winter and spring. In summer, fruits and vegetables sometimes were partially decomposed. Fresh milk also was in short supply (Fearon 1818:281; Trollope 1832a:86–87). Rancid, stale foods were common (e.g., butter and cream, and foods containing them).

In the eighteenth century, ice had been used by the very wealthy in America for cooling beverages and making ice cream, but not for general refrigeration of food. However, after the invention of the "refrigerator" (actually, an icebox) by Thomas Moore in 1803, the cooling of food became more common (Cummings 1970:36).

Ill health was rampant in the cities in the early part of the century. Epidemics of cholera, yellow fever, and typhoid raged, their causes as yet unknown. City life seemed to contribute directly to ill health. There were frequent complaints of dyspepsia (a catch-all term for stomach pains, upsets, and disorders of all kinds). In 1830, the *Encyclopedia Americana* described it as the most common of all ailments at the time (26).

Although the diets of city wage earners contained few fresh foods, it is thought that they still were better fed than their European counterparts of this era. At the close of the eighteenth century, it is said that city-dwellers rarely tasted fresh meat more than once a week (McMaster 1883:96–97). Roast beef, especially, was an infrequently consumed, but highly prized delicacy. Milk consumption continued low, particularly by modern nutrition standards. But urban workers consumed large quantities of bread. One of the cheapest sources of energy, it usually occupied the top priority in the family food budget. Potatoes also were an important staple. In New England, because wheat was expensive, the poor used corn, rye, oat and barley meals for making bread (Brayley 1909:122–24); and molasses was commonly used instead of sugar as a sweetener, since it was so much cheaper than the latter (Cummings 1970:27–9).

European travelers had regarded the diet of workers in the New World as superior to that in the Old, mainly because they perceived them to be consuming liberal amounts of meat (Cooper 1794:238). The reports were sometimes exaggerated; moreover, the meat frequently was of poor quality. Here as elsewhere in the country, during the early part of the eighteenth century the most widely used meat was salt pork. Blood pudding was a commonly consumed by-product of butchering. This food consisted of hog or occasionally beef blood, mixed with chopped pork, seasoned and stuffed in a casing. For three or four cents, a hungry worker could buy a pound of blood pudding, which, along with butter crackers, provided a meal (De Voe 1867:104–5).

Affluent Americans. Compared to the modest wage earner, the more prosperous city people enjoyed far more varied fare. Similarly, a small percentage of the American rural population—wealthy aristocrats—were able to follow a cosmopolitan menu. In contrast, most rural people enjoyed few luxuries and were consuming what must have been a bleak diet.

By this time, wealthy Americans were attempting to transcend traditional Anglo cooking, which they perceived to be lacking in elegance. According to John Adams (C.F. Adams 1876:359), the colonists had been taught by the British to dislike Parisian cookery. But French cuisine began to be popular with the fashionable following the French alliance of 1778. The first four presidents of the United States all appreciated French cuisine. In fact, Thomas Jefferson (1743–1826), the third president (1801–1809), brought a French chef to the White House. Jefferson's epicurean tastes were far-reaching and deserve some mention here. A gardener as well as a gourmet, he raised many varieties of fruits, vegetables, and herbs, both well-known and exotic. Jefferson is said to have been growing and eating tomatoes while they still were virtually unknown to most Americans. He is also credited with plying guests with such unusual delicacies as macaroni pie, ice cream served with a crust (probably a forerunner of Baked Alaska), various forms of pasta with cheese (leading to the current American staple, macaroni and cheese), a tansy (herb) pudding, and polentas (corn dishes). Jefferson undoubtedly had become acquainted with the latter during travels in southern France and northern Italy, where maize (indigenous to the western hemisphere) had become universally used by the 1780s (Crosby 1972; Jones 1990). However, despite the attraction of the affluent for French cooking, the taste for French food never entered the mainstream of American society (Levenstein 1988:11).

General Trends

Prosperous city dwellers who spent more for food than the wage earners or farmers had a more varied diet during this period. Particularly in the well-settled sections, farmers in comfortable circumstances were able to serve tasty meals, sometimes containing such delicacies as mutton, vegetables, and excellent cider (Cummings 1970:12–13).

Rancidity of foods was a common problem for Americans at all socioeconomic levels during this period, since many did not yet enjoy the use of ice for food preservation. As a result, perishable foods remained little-used luxuries, compared to the standbys of salt pork and cornmeal, which could be kept successfully throughout the year.

In the East, brown sugar and molasses (by-products of the sugar industry), along with maple syrup, were used for sweetening. However, on the plains, where these products initially were unavailable, sorghum became the common sweetener. Diets were high in fat because of the high consumption of butter, fatty cheese, and lard (Volney 1804:262). The consumption of salt (in the form of salt pork) was high. White bread (a special food for farmers) was common among the wealthy (Hale 1903:296).

Consumption of tea and coffee rose during the first three decades of the century, from about a pound per capita to about 3.5 pounds. Tea still was the more popular of the two beverages in 1800. But by 1830, coffee had become uncontested as the prime American beverage (Cummings 1970:34). This trend had begun with the onset of the Revolutionary War, when tea became politically unpopular, and later was reinforced by the War of 1812. The consumption of alcohol, mainly whiskey and other spirits, was high (chapter 10).

THE LATTER HALF OF THE NINETEENTH CENTURY (1850–1899)

This period was marked by increasing industrialization, urbanization, and modernization. As a result, the five major factors influencing food habits (physical, biological, technological, social, and cultural), as identified by Norge Jerome (1981:37) became more intricately interrelated.

Important Developments

Agricultural change. By 1850, less than 85 percent of the populace was engaged in farming or farm-related occupations. In concert with the more general Industrial Revolution, which occurred at this time, was the beginning and development of the first agriculture, food, and nutrition revolution, with its unprecedented achievements in these areas. The structure of the modern food system was established; dietary patterns began to be evaluated, and human nutrition became a popular interest. Americans began to view agriculture, food, nutrition, and commerce as an interdependent system. The events of this period were in keeping with Thomas Jefferson's belief that the nation's economic health depended on agriculture (Jerome 1981:40).

Other changes. A manufacturing boon occurred in the later 1800s, also. The Industrial Revolution and the Civil War led to a decrease in farm labor needs, with corresponding increases in movement to the cities, and migration westward.

Indian relocations. By the mid-1850s, Indian Territory included only an area almost identical with the present state of Oklahoma. It was to this region that the government moved the Choctaw, Cherokee, Chickasaw, Creek, and Seminole Indians. Known as the Five Civilized Tribes, they had lived in the Southeast, in close contact with whites, for more than 100 years. During that time, they had adopted many of the habits and customs of the whites, including the keeping of black slaves.

The Indian Territory had no uniform political organization. The Indians were permitted to govern themselves as long as they kept the peace. In 1866, the tribes were required to give up the western part of their territory to the United States for the use of other Indians. This was partly to punish them for helping the South during the Civil War. Some of the lands in this region not assigned as Indian reservations were opened up to white settlement in 1889. So many white settlers came in that the Territory of Oklahoma in the western part of the present State of Oklahoma was organized during the following year.

Food-related Developments

Developments initiated during the early years of the nineteenth century now resulted in significant changes in food production, storage, preservation, and marketing with a significant impact on the diet.

New knowledge within the agriculture sciences, along with new technologies, were being applied to farming practices. After 1850, farms were mechanized rapidly. Better tools, along with farm mechanization and specialization and fertilization, all combined to bring about great improvements in American agriculture. These advances, along with the increased use of business methods by farmers, significantly increased the supply of food. Additional factors further expanded the distribution of both land and food. These included continued immigration, pertinent legislation, especially the Homestead Act and the Morrill Act (both in 1862); the coming of railroads, and the development of canning.

Immigration. During the first century of U.S. history, only about 10,000 new settlers had arrived yearly. However, by the 1830s, immigration began to increase appreciably. The period 1830–60 is known as the "first wave of immigration" (Rischin 1989) (see table 5.1). During the decades of 1830, 1840, and 1850, the number of immigrants rose from 600,000 to 1.7 million and 2.6 million, respectively. Most of these new residents were from Germany, Great Britain and, especially, Ireland. The latter had suffered severe famines due to failure of their potato crop caused by potato blight. The potato had become a staple in Ireland, following its introduction from the New World in the sixteenth century. Following a widespread failure of the potato crop in 1845 and 1846, nearly a fifth of the Irish population died. Many of the survivors fled to America. Because of their bitter experience with crop raising, few of the Irish went west, unlike the Germans. Instead, they settled in the urban areas of the East. By 1910, 4 of the 25 million inhabitants of the United States were Irish. Thus, a distant potato famine thoroughly changed the population and political face of many American cities.

The Homestead Act of 1862, with its promise of land, attracted many who were interested in farming, triggering the second wave of immigrants, who arrived between 1860 and 1890. The largest proportion of these people were from Germany, Great Britain, Ireland, and the Scandinavian nations. Gradually, the newcomers came mainly from Austria-Hungary, Italy, and Russia.

Between 1890 and 1930, the third wave of immigrants came, which exceeded the total from colonial times until then (table 5.1). They were mostly from Greece, Hungary, Italy, Poland, Portugal, Russia, and Spain. The government began to restrict immigration in 1882.

Morrill Act. This act, passed in 1862 by the Congress under President Abraham Lincoln, granted that the proceeds from federally owned lands be used for perpetual endowment of Land Grant colleges. These colleges were directed to offer instruction in agriculture and the mechanical arts, which included home economics. These colleges, most of which later became universities, were directed to teach, to do research, and to take knowledge to the people. This mandate resulted in the development of many extension programs, aimed at the dissemination of information to farmers and other groups within the population. Many people credit the bounty of the U.S. food supply to the increases in food production made possible by the Agricultural Experiment Stations and Land Grant universities in every state of the union.

Transportation. The coming of railroads was very important to the food industry because it enabled the shipment of fresh eggs, meat, milk, and fresh produce to cities throughout the Eastern seaboard. The first transcontinental railroad, the Union Pacific, was completed in 1869, opening up the West and allowing the transportation of food and other products from coast to coast.

Food preservation. The invention of a simple canning process by Nicholas Appert, a French chef, in 1809, led to the development of the canning industry. In 1859, the Mason jar was perfected. The Civil War served as a powerful impetus to the canning industry, because of the great need for canned foods to feed the soldiers. With the development of the Mason jar, and large pressure cookers (called retorts) in 1874, canning emerged as a form of food preservation, both at the home (in kitchens, such as the one shown in Figure 5.3) and factory levels. Pioneers in food preservation include the Underwood family of Boston, who produced canned seafoods and meats, including a line of highly seasoned ("deviled") canned meat products for sandwich spreads (Figure 5.4). Lyman Underwood and Dr. Samuel Prescott of the Massachusetts Institute of Technology are well known for their landmark cooperative research near the end of the century on spoilage in canned foods. In 1875, both Gustavus F. Swift and P. D. Armour established their famous meatpacking plants in Chicago.

Jerome (1981:40) has observed that two major developments during this period—the introduction of the refrigerated railroad car in 1870, and the development of the pressure cooker in 1874—transformed the preservation, storage, and distribution of foods.

Food laws. Legal attempts to improve food are illustrated by an 1850 Massachusetts law prohibiting the adulteration of milk. Milk was sold in bottles in the late 1850s in Brooklyn; bottling and the concept of certified milk, for which the medical milk commissions set up standards, were further efforts to produce and sell safe milk. Dr. Harvey Wiley, who was the prime mover in the enactment of federal pure food and drug legislation, became chief of the Chemical Division of the U.S. Department of Agriculture in 1883. These are only a few of the early efforts that have developed into the present system of safeguarding the U.S. food supply.

Eating Patterns of the Period

Industrialization and urbanization during the first half of the nineteenth century had resulted in a prosperous and expanding middle class. This segment became much more firmly established after the outbreak of the Civil War in 1861. It is to this affluent and status-conscious tier of Amer-

Figure 5.3
Kitchen, 1874

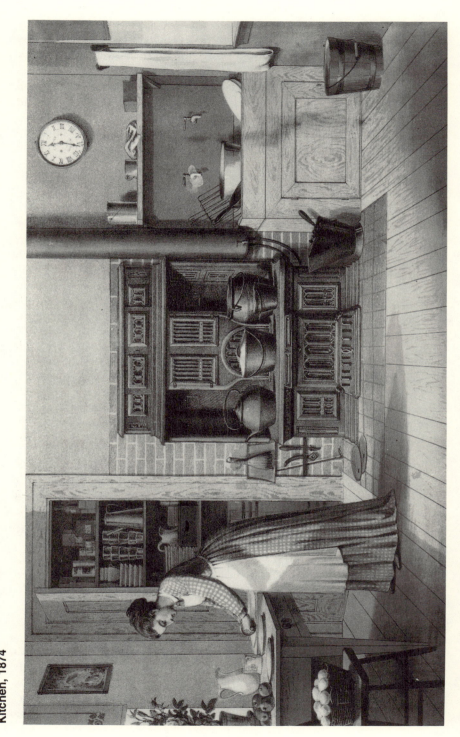

Lithograph by L. Prang & Company. Courtesy of the Library of Congress.

Figure 5.4
Original Underwood® Deviled Canned Product Trademark

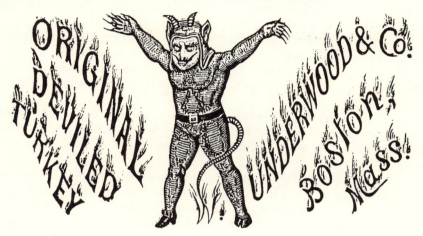

TRADE-MARK.
——o——
W. J. UNDERWOOD.

(No. 2,297. Registered March 16, 1875.)

DEVILED ENTREMETS.

No. 10,051.   Registered Feb. 13, 1883

This Red Devil trademark, first used in 1867, is the oldest registered trademark in use in the United States. Courtesy of Pet Incorporated.

ican society that historians have accorded the most visibility. However, by far the greatest number of Americans at this time, both rural and urban, were making only a modest living. For others, such as the poor sharecroppers and city wage earners, simply obtaining enough to eat was still an ongoing challenge. City workers were at the bottom of the economic ladder and most at risk nutritionally.

Rural population. People in the rural sectors had the advantage of being able to grow most of their own food. By the last half of the century, there was more emphasis on the raising of vegetables in the rural sectors than during pioneer days. People had become more aware of the need for vegetables in the diet. The rise in market gardening, particularly on farms near urban areas, may have provided additional stimulus.

Unfortunately, "hog 'n' hominy" still was the chief fare in the southern and western communities not yet serviced by railroads. According to Frederick Law Olmsted, who traveled during the 1850s throughout the South, southern planters subsisted mainly on bacon (sometimes cooked with turnip greens), corn pone, and coffee sweetened with molasses (Olmsted 1857: 15; 1860:396). Slaves generally fared better, because they usually kept gardens that provided vegetables.

After 1870, both rural and urban homemakers were taking up canning as a way of providing their families with a supply of fruits and vegetables for the winter. Rural housewives tended to put up foods from their own gardens while urban homemakers could purchase quantities of foods in season from local markets.

With the trend away from open pasturage, the building of dairy barns, and putting up of hay and fodder for the winter, milk now was being produced the year around. Farm families, especially, were drinking more milk.

Urban population. With the coming of railroads, perishable foods now were available in much more ample supply in the large cities. The refrigerated box car soon assured the delivery of fresh milk, fruits, and vegetables. However, the diets of middle- and upper-class people in the large cities benefited the most from these advances, since they could afford to purchase those foods which had become available.

In the smaller towns, the diets were still markedly seasonal until the turn of the century. Customarily, there was a lack of fresh fruit, except apples, and there were no green vegetables in the winter (Levenstein 1988:25; Lynd and Lynd 1929:157–58).

Senator Albert J. Beveridge from Indiana gave Morison this description of the breakfasting habits of the people in his native village in Indiana before the Civil War:

> Shortly after dawn the men might be seen issuing from their cabins and houses, converging on the village butcher's, where each purchased a beefsteak cut from an animal slaughtered the previous evening. Coming and going, they stopped at the village store for a dram of corn whiskey. Returning, their wives prepared a breakfast of black coffee, fried beefsteak, and hot cornbread. (Morison 1965:473)

After 1840, urban food costs in relation to wages fell greatly. By the 1850s and 1860s workers were buying more lean meat, milk, leafy vegetables, and fruit. The exception was during the Civil War, when fresh meat became so costly, workers could afford only a "half ration." Although the daily per capita consumption of milk had been rising modestly since 1833, by 1864, at ⅓ of a pint, it was still barely enough to use for one's coffee or for one's oatmeal at breakfast (Cummings 1970:77). Unfortunately, the aftermath of the Civil War did not bring about general dietary improvements. During the 1870s, the economy was not good. As a result, there were grave effects on employment and wages among the new working class (Levenstein 1988:44). Emancipated slaves were experiencing tremendous adjustments as they began new lives. Freedom meant trading the relative security of the plantations for riskier ventures, such as becoming sharecoppers or migrating to the cities, where finding employment often was a problem. In either case, they usually stopped raising gardens. Consequently, over the short term, the general quality of their diets suffered.

General Dietary Trends

The dietary pattern of this era has been described as follows by Calla Van Syckle:

The basic standard for the American table—the standard toward which families moved as soon as economic conditions or technological developments permitted—remained the same up to 1900. It included meat in relatively large quantities, with beef predominating and pork second in popularity; potatoes, cabbage, onions, and other fresh vegetables in season and in moderate amounts; a variety of fresh fruits in summer but chiefly apples in winter; white bread and rolls, cakes and pies; butter, eggs, milk for baking and relatively moderate or small amounts for drinking; preserves, coffee and tea. A diet high in meats, sweets, and white flour foods represented a traditionally high standard of living to the emigrants from the British Isles, Ireland, Northern Europeans and Scandinavian countries who made up the bulk of our population. (1945b:690)

Middle class. As can be inferred from the foregoing description, the solid middle class had entered an era of abundance. As soon as their economic status permitted, Americans typically began to buy beef. Although it was more popular than pork, it should be noted that far more pork than beef still was being consumed nationwide. This trend began in early colonial times and continued for 300 years.

Upper class. Although the national cuisine during this period was abundant, the wealthy found it lacking in elegance. Therefore, it intensified its preoccupation with European (especially French) cuisine, which had begun in the early years of the nineteenth century. However, this enthusiasm for French cuisine was never shared by the mainstream of American society.

Victorian age. This period came to full flower during the last half of the nineteenth century, when a new class of Americans emerged, the Victorian middle class. Susan Williams (1985:1) has characterized this group as "proper and prosperous." However, the boundaries of this new class were constantly shifting, creating an unsettling degree of social uncertainty. Americans responded by meticulously observing the rules of etiquette to demonstrate and maintain their newly won place in society. Thus, dining rituals—how they ate; the dining room furniture, decorations, and table settings; how they dressed for dinner; and the menus chosen—became very important. To middle-class Victorians, dining habits provided visible reassurance of their established and secure social position within a changing world (ix) (Figure 5.5).

For these reasons, well-to-do Americans during this period frequently entertained friends and associates at elaborate, multicourse dinner parties at well-appointed tables, attended by servants. However, informal family meals were much simpler.

In more modest homes, dinner was often less a gathering for society than a gathering for sustenance. Many American tables were covered with white oilcloth, rather than damask, and supper, under fortunate circumstances, might include butter, jam, or condensed milk for the children to spread on their bread, or cheese and a pint of beer for the adults (Williams 1985:4).

In the extremely class-conscious society of the post–Civil War era, Americans of means seemed to pattern their meals slavishly after overly mannered and pretentious European models (Williams 1985:5). However, despite a deep-seated and anxious interest in "civilization" (usually denoting European), Americans also shared a special regard for their own unique history and past. The latter served as a careful ideological control during the evolution of a national self-image, particularly in the dining room. "While Americans continued to look to their European past for refinement, they selectively scrutinized their own colonial past for evidence of moral supremacy, national mettle, and personal ingenuity. Thus 'civilization' for them increasingly became an amalgam of anything from the past, be it European or distinctively American, that proved useful in ordering their increasingly complex world" (10).

Williams has observed that "by the end of the nineteenth century, the colonial past was generally revered through a special brand of nostalgia keynoted in colonial furnishings, dwellings, modes of behavior, and cultural vigor; and the ruder, less stylized aspects of those days were carefully forgotten" (10). (As in all societies, it is the eating habits of the rich which have been the best documented.)

OVERVIEW

The nineteenth century serves as an excellent illustration of how food habits change in response to social developments such as increasing population diversity, the growth of cities, and technical developments such as refrigeration, improved transportation, and the processing of foods.

In the light of current nutrition knowledge, many people within both the rural and urban sectors suffered from serious dietary deficiencies during the early years of the republic (1789–1850). Generally, the consumption of the perishable foods (milk, fresh fruits, and vegetables, as well as fresh meats) was inadequate. Urban workers and their families were less well fed than the rural population, because they could raise little if any of their own food and had limited resources with which to buy what foods were available in

Figure 5.5
Dining Room, 1890s

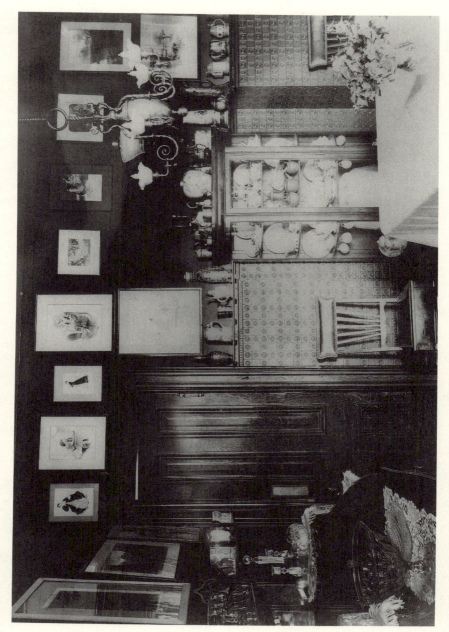

the city during this era. The nutritional status of blacks was much the same as it had been during the colonial period, since most of them were still kept on plantations at this time. Many Indians had been uprooted as a result of the Indian Removal Act of 1830, with its subsequent relocations. Thousands of Indians had died because of disease and malnutrition associated with these circumstances.

Lack of fruits and vegetables (along with inadequate milk consumption) led to deficiencies in numerous vitamins and minerals necessary for proper growth and maintenance of the body. These included vitamin C, riboflavin, calcium, and vitamins A and D. All of the dietary faults of the period cited here surely must have contributed to the generally low life expectancy and smaller stature of Americans during this period.

Generally, Americans' milk consumption, as well as their intake of fruits and vegetables increased during the last half of the nineteenth century. Their better total nutrition is saliently demonstrated by the fact that Americans were increasing in both size and girth, and living longer.

FOR FURTHER READING

Cummings, R.O. 1970. *The American and his food* (rev. ed.). New York: Arno Press.

Dick, E. 1937. *The sod-house frontier, 1854–1890*. New York: D. Appleton-Century Company.

Grover, K. (ed.). 1987. *Dining in America, 1850–1900*. Amherst: University of Massachusetts Press and Rochester, New York: Margaret Woodbury Strong Museum.

Jerome, N.W. 1981. The U.S. dietary pattern from an anthropological perspective. *Food Technology* 35(2):37–42.

Levenstein, H.A. 1988. *Revolution at the table*. New York: Oxford University Press.

Lowenberg, M.E., E.N. Todhunter, E.D. Wilson, J.R. Savage, and J.L. Lubawski. 1979. *Food and people* (3rd ed.). New York: John Wiley and Sons.

Morison, S.E. 1965. *The Oxford history of the American people*. New York: Oxford University Press.

Root, W., and R. de Rochemont. 1976. *Eating in America*. New York: Ecco Press.

Van Syckle, C. 1945a. Pictures of food consumption in the United States: Part I, 1630–1860. *J. Am. Diet. Assoc.* 19:508–12.

———. 1945b. Some pictures of food consumption in the United States: Part II, 1860–1941. *J. Am. Diet. Assoc.* 21:690–95.

Williams, S. 1985. *Savory suppers and fashionable feasts*. New York: Pantheon Books.

6

American Food Habits: The Twentieth Century

THE FIRST AGRICULTURAL REVOLUTION EXPANDS (1900–1920)

The first two decades of the twentieth century marked the expansion of industrialized agriculture, which had begun in 1850 (chapter 4). Increased mechanization and industrialization had a far-reaching, positive effect on the food system of the United States. In addition to increasing food production, these forces effected changes in food processing, transportation, and distribution of food as well.

Farmers were becoming increasingly mechanized, with positive effects on food production. Steam-powered implements, used by some farmers in the nineteenth century, were being used more widely (Figure 6.1). Later, they began to be replaced by those which were gasoline powered. By the early 1900s, engineers had designed gasoline-powered tractors powerful enough to pull a plow. However, horses still remained important for farm work.

By 1900, improved, more efficient farming methods had encouraged the increased migration of people to the city, because fewer farm workers were needed. This trend, coupled with a sharply increased influx of immigrants (Jenks and Lauck 1926), most of whom now were choosing to locate in America's cities and industrial towns, resulted in a country that was by now, only 60 percent rural. Many factors, working together, stimulated the food industry during the early 1900s. The increase in both the size and

Figure 6.1
Threshing Grain Using Steam Engine, 1900

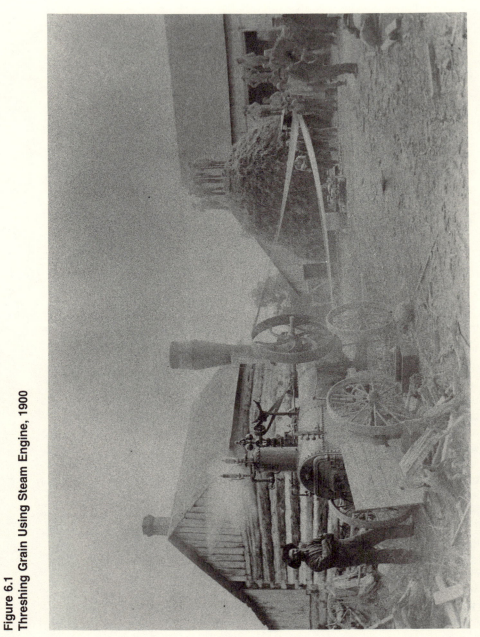

heterogeneity of the population, along with increased urbanization, all changed the social environment, creating additional demands for more food, both in quantity and diversity. A prime triumph of twentieth century America is that its food system was able to respond successfully to this challenge.

Food-related Developments

Railroad cars were transporting food regularly to consumers. Refrigerated cars were especially valuable for the perishable foods: fresh fruits and vegetables, meats, dairy products, and eggs. The icebox still was the only form of home refrigeration during this period (Figure 5.2). In 1903, agricultural scientists made an indelible impact on the modern American diet with the development of "iceberg lettuce," which was very hardy and held up well during shipping and storage (Williams 1985:14).

Techniques such as the Mason jar and the Shriver pressure cooker, or retort, introduced in the nineteenth century, now were used widely. Food processing became increasingly commonplace, both in factories and in homes, so that people no longer were restricted to eating seasonal foods (Figure 6.2). By 1900, the American food-processing industry already had become big business, accounting for 20 percent of the nation's manufacturing. The main food sectors already were dominated by a few giant corporations. Increased mechanization of food preparation and improvements in canning technology greatly increased the productivity of canners. By 1910, ten years before the real heyday of American canning, more than 68,000 people turned out over 3 billion cans of food (Hampe and Wittenberg 1964; Levenstein 1988).

Food safety. Along with increased availability of foods, developments during this period also led to increased safety of the food supply. Since the late nineteenth century, there had been growing concern on the part of consumers regarding the healthfulness of their food. The conditions under which food was processed and marketed were often unsanitary; spoilage was common, and unsafe ingredients frequently were added.

A drive for meat inspection, which had begun in the 1880s, led to the passage of a federal meat inspection law in 1891. It was followed by the new, tougher federal Meat Inspection Act of 1906.

Dr. Harvey Wiley, chief chemist of the U.S. Department of Agriculture, was a leading crusader in the movement to obtain federal regulation of food additives and compulsory labeling of ingredients. The efforts of this movement culminated in the enactment in 1906 of the Pure Food and Drug Act. This law has been described as the most significant peacetime legislation in the history of the country (Hill 1964).

In 1908, concern over the purity of milk led to the enactment of the first

Figure 6.2
Cheese Factory, 1910–1915

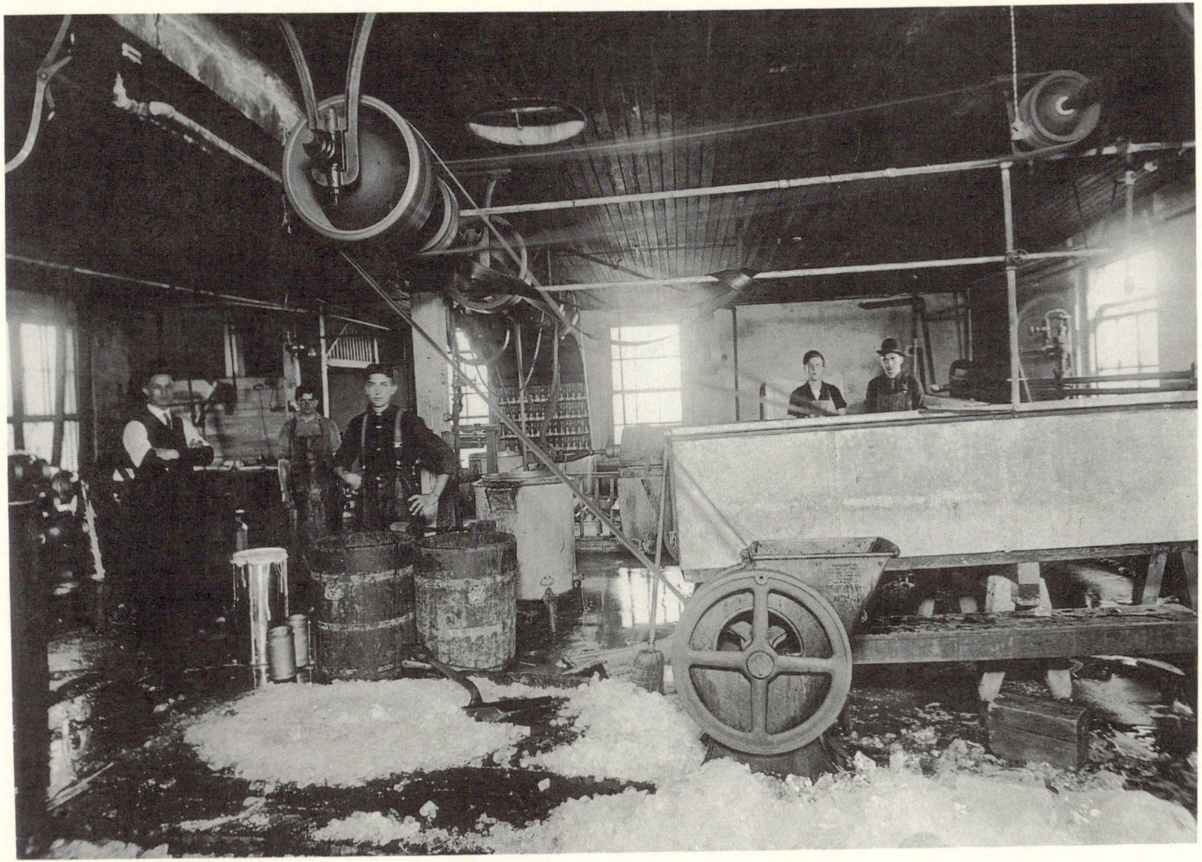

Food processing became increasingly common during the early 1900s. The Neville Public Museum of Brown County.

compulsory pasteurization law, in Chicago. By 1920, many similar laws had been passed at local and state levels, requiring the pasteurization of milk.

All of these regulations led to the consolidation of the milk, meat, and food-processing industries. Giant corporations replaced the many smaller companies who could not afford the investments necessary for the equipment and monitoring required to comply with the new "pure food laws." The names Nabisco (National Biscuit Company), Heinz, Van Camp's, and Campbell Soup were well known, as well as the names of the Big Five in meatpacking (Armour, Swift, Wilson, Morris, and Cudahy) (Ross 1980).

Food, nutrition, and World War I. The United States entered World War I in April 1917. Shortly thereafter, Herbert Hoover was appointed to head the newly authorized U.S. Food Administration and was given broad powers over the prices, production, and distribution of food. The central strategy of the Food Administration (FA), which actually had been conceived during the food crisis of the winter of 1916–17, was one of voluntary restriction of white wheat flour, meat, sugar, and butter. In addition to occasional calls for general reductions in food consumption, "wheatless" and "meatless" days were promoted, based on the basic concept of substitutions set forth by Wilbur Atwater, the noted American nutritionist, and his followers. Americans were reminded of Atwater's teachings that they could obtain proteins, fats, and carbohydrates from diverse, not necessarily expensive, food sources (Atwater 1887; 1888a). By way of applying these concepts, they were urged to get their protein from beans rather than meat, their carbohydrates from cornmeal, oats, and grains other that wheat, and their fats from lard and vegetable oils. Home economists, recruited for the FA effort, devised recipes and menus that would employ substitutes for wheat, beef, butter, and sugar. Italian immigrants provided practical meatless or meat-conserving recipes involving pasta and tomato sauce, which became increasingly popular during the 1920s. Thus, Italian food became the first immigrant food to gain widespread acceptance. Since fruits and vegetables were too perishable to send to Europe, their consumption was encouraged, an unexpected nutritional boon for the American public. Although the Food Administration's efforts had their greatest impact on the middle and upper classes, their importance should not be underestimated. Certainly, they had a significant influence on food habits and ideas, encouraging Americans to consider more seriously what and how much they were eating (Levenstein 1988).

Eating Patterns of the Period

What did Americans of the early 1900s eat? Except for the very poor, who had insufficient money to buy food, most people ate more food than necessary; obesity and digestive problems related to overeating were common. Both upper and lower classes tended to overeat, albeit for different reasons. The upper class tended to overeat because their affluence afforded them a wide selection of food and drink, while the lower classes might overeat in part because they were likely to be doing hard physical labor. Drinking was heavy, particularly among the working class.

First generation immigrants were especially focused on food, since food scarcity often had been the prime motivation for their immigration to America in the first place. Generally, diet contained much more meat than was necessary for adequate protein intake, and certainly more meat than these people had been accustomed to eating back in their native lands. Pork, which initially had been America's prime animal meat source, still remained the country's most common meat three centuries later (Root and de Rochemont 1976). By the 1900s, frowned on by the nutritionists of the day (probably because of its fat content), pork began to lose popularity with the upper class. However, it continued to occupy an important place in the American diet, particularly for factory workers, midwesterners, and southerners.

Rural population. The diets of rural Americans varied widely, depending in large part on their economic well-being. Tenant farmers and sharecroppers were especially likely to have an inadequate diet, since they usually were forced to raise cash crops to the exclusion of garden foods, meats, and poultry for their tables. Pellagra was common. By contrast, the better-off farmers, particularly those who owned their own farms and produced most of their own food, often had diets that included a wide variety of nutritious foods.

Urban population. After 1900, immigration increased dramatically. Between 1901 and 1910, 1 million new immigrants arrived, mainly from central and southern Europe, including large numbers of Italians, Jews, and Poles. Most of these new immigrants gravitated to the cities and industrial towns (Jenks and Lauck 1926).

Beginning in the 1880s, a bilevel working class had developed, consisting of the relatively well-off skilled and semiskilled and the struggling, unskilled workers. After 1900, this division became reinforced by ethnic differences, since most of the new immigrants were in the latter category. In contrast, the upper sector consisted mainly of native born or first generation people of Anglo-Saxon and northern European origin. These two groups observed different eating patterns, reflecting their differing cultural and geographical origins, as well as economic status (Levenstein 1988). However, for every working man, bread, potatoes, cabbage, and onions were essential items in the diet. Fortuitously, both potatoes and cabbage (often called the poor man's sources of vitamin C) provided much-needed ascorbic acid. The more skilled workers, mainly with origins in the British Isles, tended to follow typical "New England cuisine," which had developed during colonial days (chapter 4), or modifications thereof.

Figure 6.3
Grocery Store in Kansas, c. 1900

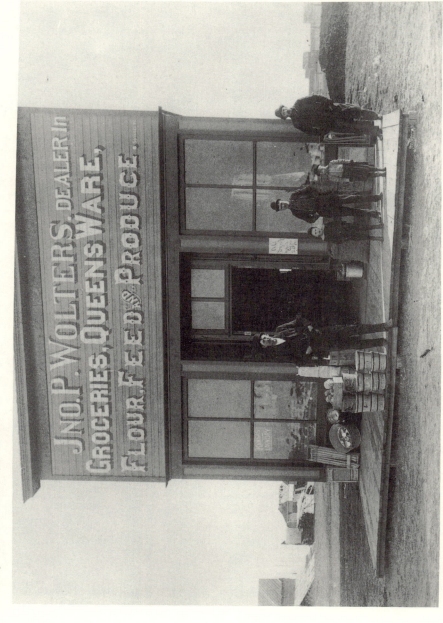

Figure 6.4
Kitchen/Bedroom of New York City Tenement, 1900s

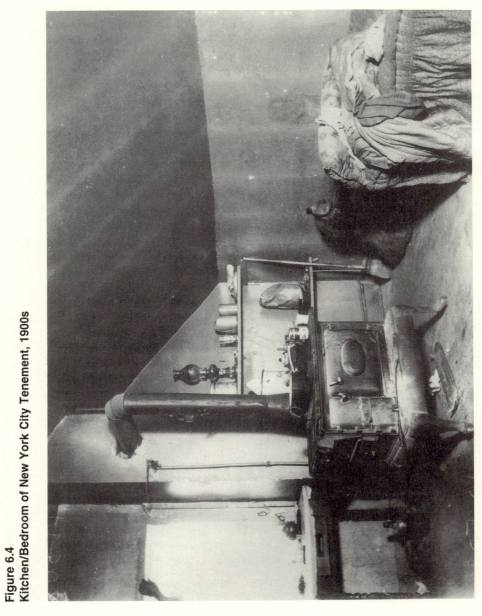

The diets of the skilled or semiskilled workers were liberal and varied, clearly reflective of their relative prosperity and the good selection of foods now available. These workers' meals included fresh meat of all kinds, eggs, potatoes, white sauce, fruits and vegetables (particularly the canned variety), as well as desserts (including the proverbial apple pie).

The "new immigrants" were fond of "multifood dishes" such as stews, goulashes, and Italian pasta/tomatoes/sausage, which were frowned on by the native-born Americans and, surprisingly, even the home economists of the day. The latter believed that foods mixed together were not assimilated as well as those served separately. (Obviously, professionals of the time did not take into account the fact that all foods, when taken in the same meal, become mixtures in the stomach upon ingestion.)

Most of the immigrants came from cultures in which bread had been a much-depended-on staple of symbolic significance. It remained an essential component of their diets in the United States, usually purchased from ethnic bakeries where breads exactly like those eaten in the old countries were available. The new immigrants preferred bread, coffee, and often soup for their breakfasts.

While more affluent families used commercially canned fruits and vegetables (a symbol of Americanization), immigrant women relied mainly on home canning—preserving quantities of fruit and vegetables in the summer and fall—for their families' meals in the off-season (Levenstein 1988). Workers' expenditures for food in 1918 consumed close to 40 percent of their budgets (Douglas 1930).

Middle class. By 1900, nutritionists were focusing much of their energies toward changing the diet of the middle class. Efforts of the "nutrition reformers" of the 1890s to reach the poor urban factory worker had failed. And the nutrition message preached by Atwater and his followers during the 1890s, that of getting better nutrition by eating less, was far from being taken seriously by most Americans. But many members of the middle class (better educated, and more impressed with the scientific approach) were attracted to Atwater's nutrition teachings.

With their new interest and concerns for health and nutrition, the middle class of Americans became vulnerable to all sorts of food fads and quackery during the early decades of the twentieth century. This interest stemmed in part from various physical disorders, commonly experienced during this time by those individuals whose comfortable circumstances enabled them to indulge in overeating and overdrinking.

Fortunately, not all of the food fads explored by Americans during this period were nutritionally bad. One dietary innovation that had a valid nutritional rationale was the use of dried commercial breakfast cereals. By the 1900s, although meat continued to occupy a prime place in the general American diet, the leading breakfast food pioneers (William R. Kellogg and Charles W. Post, in particular) succeeded in promoting various cereal products as substitutes for the traditional meats typically consumed at breakfast. These entrepreneurs emphasized the health advantages of this recommended dietary change. Their promotional strategy was tremendously effective, in part because, by the turn of the century, the middle class had become very concerned about the relationship between food and health.

Middle-class dining. During the years following 1880, the middle class had expanded considerably, along with industrialization and urbanization. By the early 1900s, blessed with rising economic status and the ready availability of foods (both imported and domestic), it was becoming increasingly desirous of adopting the dining styles of the upper class. Ultimately, however, the problems in obtaining satisfactory domestic service, the warnings of nutritionists against overeating, and the underlying desire of middle-class women to reduce the hours spent in the kitchen all contributed to a change in what American society expected of middle-class cuisine, both in quantity and quality. After 1905, there was a definite shift toward smaller and less elaborate meals. Labor was saved by simpler menus, fewer ingredients in dishes, fewer steps in their preparation, and fewer courses. It was through their role in effecting these changed expectations that the home economists of the day had their greatest influence on middle-class foodways (Levenstein 1988).

CRISIS YEARS, 1920–1940

The character of this period was shaped strongly by two major crises— the Great Depression and the drought of the 1930s. Except for a year or two at the beginning of the decade, the 1920s were a prosperous period for business. However, most farms were beset with economic problems. Prices for farm products fell about 40 percent in 1920 and 1921, and remained low through the 1920s. Many farmers lost their farms through bankruptcy and were forced to become renters or to abandon farming.

The stock market crash of October 29, 1929, heralded the Great Depression, a worldwide business slump that continued through the 1930s. It was the worst and longest period of high unemployment and low business activity in modern times. Adding to the gravity of the situation were the severe droughts, dust storms, and erosion that hit parts of the Midwest and Southwest during the 1930s. The most severe droughts occurred in 1934 and 1936. Thousands of farmers were wiped out, many of whom migrated to the fertile agricultural areas of California, hoping to find work. Most of those who found jobs had to work as fruit pickers for extremely low wages. The migrant families crowded into shacks near the fields or camped outdoors. The experiences of typical migrant families are described vividly by John Steinbeck (1939) in his novel *The Grapes of Wrath.*

Federalism. The period between the stock market crash in October 1929, and March 1933, when Franklin Delano Roosevelt (FDR) became presi-

Figure 6.5
Farmer Separating Cream from Milk, 1920s

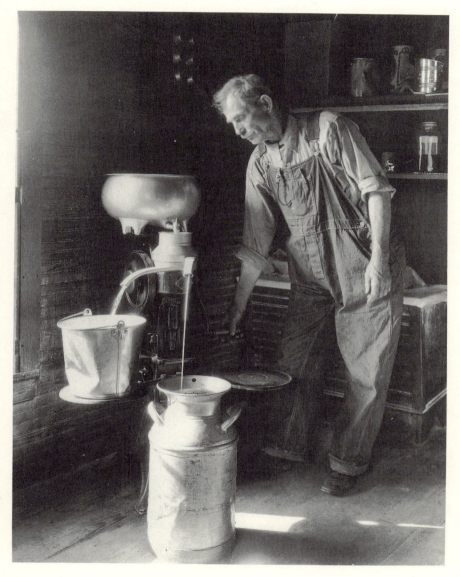

Photographed by G. Ackerman. United States Department of Agriculture (USDA).

dent, marked the worst of the Great Depression in the United States. FDR's first term as president saw the beginning of twentieth-century federalism in the United States. Upon taking office, Roosevelt immediately called Congress into special session to pass laws to alleviate the depression, naming his program the New Deal. Many agencies (sometimes called alphabet soup) evolved from this legislation, designed to manage relief and recovery programs. The establishment of such agencies as the Civilian Conservation Corps (CCC) and the Public Works Administration (PWA) in 1933 and the Works Progress Administration (WPA) in 1935 provided employment for thousands of people.

During the 1930s, the government became intimately involved with America's food system as it responded to the dual crises of depression and drought. It launched numerous efforts to safeguard the nation's agricultural base. Nonetheless, millions of small farmers were forced to abandon their farms and migrate to urban areas. The low prices for farm products, which had existed since the early 1920s, finally drove many farmers to dump milk, shoot cattle, and burn grains for fuel, rather than sell them for nothing. In an attempt to remedy this dilemma, price supports were authorized and, for the first time, the federal government began to buy farm products directly (Schlossberg 1978). Other important legislation included the Agricultural Adjustment Act of 1933 and the Social Security Act of 1935. The long drought, exacerbated by unwise farming techniques, led to serious erosion and the subsequent loss of good soil. Concern for this threat to America's farmland led to the establishment, in 1939, of the Soil Conservation Service, a government agency within the United States Department of Agriculture (USDA).

Food-related Developments

Refrigeration. During the 1920s mechanical refrigerators became available for those who could afford them. However, a model kitchen in 1924 does not yet show one (Figure 6.6).

Malnutrition. Malnutrition smoldered during the 1930s, affecting both urban and rural Americans. It had its greatest impact on such target groups as dwellers in the urban ghetto, the rural poor, migrant workers, and Native Americans. However, malnutrition also touched large numbers of the middle class, who were left jobless by the depression.

Food subsidies. The Roosevelt administration authorized two food subsidy programs under the commodity food legislation in 1935. These programs distributed surplus agricultural products to families and to schools, respectively. The commodity products included canned meat and poultry, dried beans, canned fruits and vegetables, cooking and eating fats, cornmeal, flour, nonfat dried milk, peanut butter, rice, rolled wheat, and other cereals. These foods provided essential supplemental nutrition to the diets

Figure 6.6
Model Kitchen, 1924

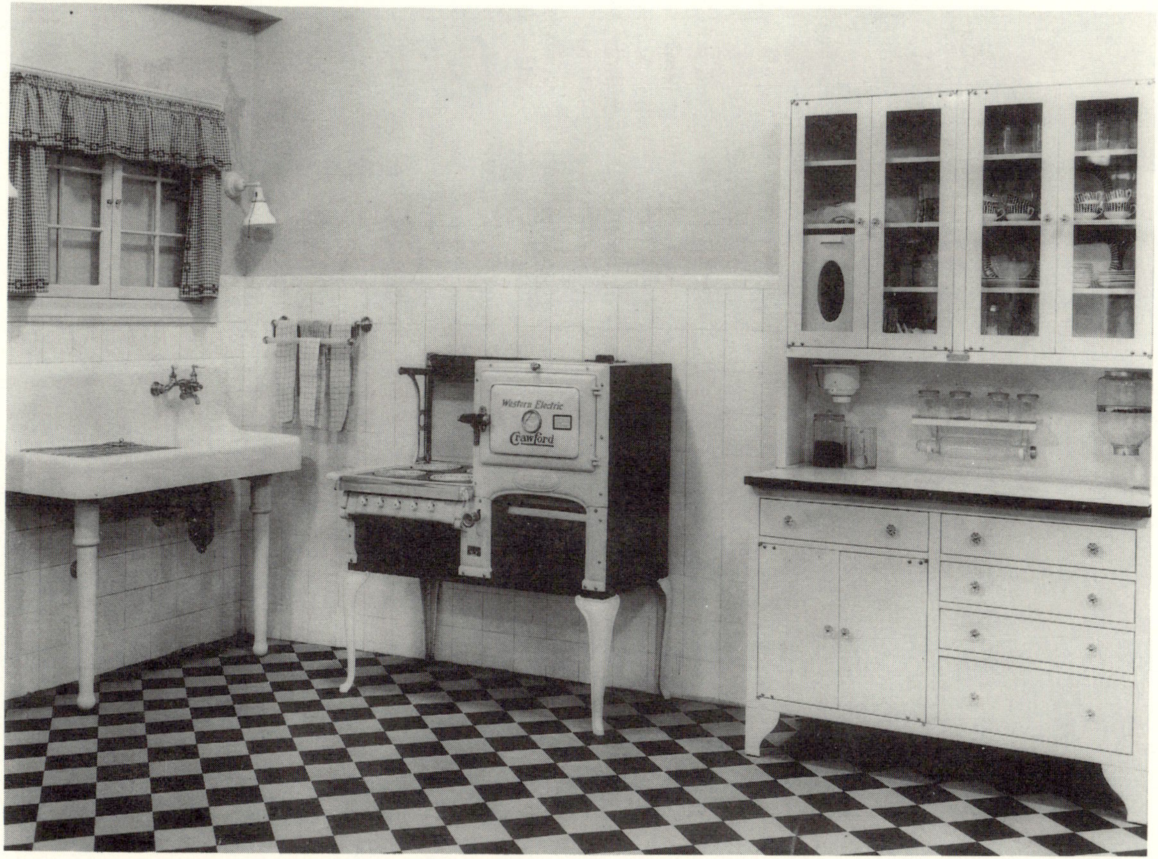

of many families and children. The commodity food programs proved to be forerunners of stronger, expanded programs which still continue today: School Lunch (1946) and the Commodity Distribution Program (1949).

Food safety. By the 1930s, the original Food and Drug Act had become inadequate because of the increased complexity and breadth of the food system. In response to increased needs and consumer pressure, the federal Food, Drug, and Cosmetic Act was enacted in 1938.

Eating Patterns of the Period

Rural population. Poor diets were not uncommon in the rural areas of America. Tenants and sharecroppers in the South (both blacks and whites) were still consuming a diet consisting mainly of the "3 M's" (maize, molasses, and meat [meaning salt pork, which was almost all fat and no lean]), and outbreaks of pellagra remained common. Pressure to produce cash crops rendered it virtually impossible for them to raise the garden crops and domestic animals that would have provided the fresh produce, meat, and milk so needed to augment their diets. Poor nutrition also was common amongst the mountain people of Appalachia, who consumed similar diets.

Urban population. A 1924 study of more than 12,000 families in 42 states (the largest survey of the decade) by the Bureau of Labor Statistics, showed that, on average, over 38 percent of worker's expenditures still went for food. This figure was similar to that of Douglas (1930), who calculated that workers' budgets for food dropped from 43.1 percent in 1901 to 38.2 percent in 1918. The most important changes took place in how the food dollar now was spent and what it bought. The cost of key items in the workers' budget, such as flour, potatoes, and some meats, decreased substantially or stabilized at a relatively low level. Income was thus freed up for the purchase of more fruits and vegetables, whose prices remained about the same (U.S. Bureau of the Census 1975). New York City workers in 1928 showed similar levels of meat consumption, but lower prices, and a larger percent for milk, cheese, fruits and vegetables. They ate less flour and cereals, and, as income increased, more meats and grains. Their diets, by 1930s standards, were judged to be much healthier than in 1914 (Gillett and Rice 1931).

Diet and low economic status. The working class still was much too concerned about obtaining adequate food to become very involved with the calorie-counting and dieting in vogue with the middle class during this period. For many workers, the prime problem still was simply getting enough to eat.

Although, in general, the economic status of urban workers improved during the 1920s, at least one in 10 workers was unemployed at any given time during this period (Bernstein 1970). An urban underclass seemed to be emerging, which included blacks who had been migrating from the rural

Figure 6.7
Farmer's Market at Washington and Reade Streets, New York City, 1929

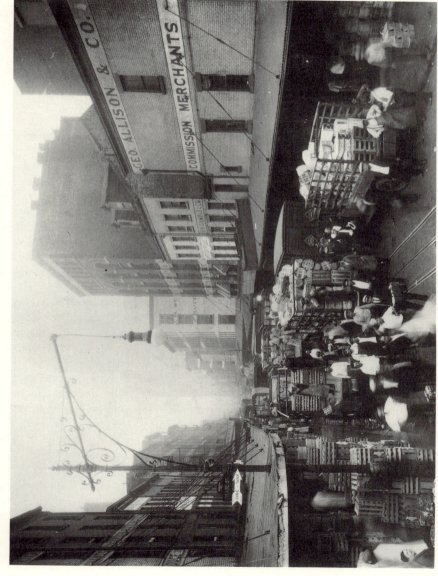

United States Department of Agriculture (USDA)

South to industrial cities in the North and Midwest. In their new environment, they tended to retain the salt pork and corn of their traditional diets, adding white flour, sweets, and highly processed foods now available to them, but little milk and fresh fruits and vegetables. The result was a nutritionally inadequate diet, frequently inferior to that of the slave (chapter 4). Poor diet undoubtedly contributed to their high infant mortality rate, twice that of the urban whites (Jones 1985; Kessler-Harris 1982). However, by the 1930s, low-income persons were benefiting greatly from the surplus foods available to them through the Commodity Food Program.

Americanization effects. Ethnic eating habits were becoming Americanized. The Immigration Act of 1924 seriously curtailed further immigration from southern and eastern Europe, which previously had provided periodic arrivals of newcomers, bringing fresh reinforcement of old country foodways. First generation immigrants also were influenced by their children, who brought home American ideas gained from their outside contacts (e.g., school home economics courses, school lunch programs, women's magazines, and movies). Second generation immigrants tended to be especially desirous of abandoning old country food habits. Increasingly, immigrant families began to use dry breakfast cereals, canned goods, and other typically American prepared foods.

Middle class. During this period, there was a growing desire for lessened household labor (a result of many factors, including woman suffrage and the generally expanding outside interests of women). This motive, along with a preoccupation with dieting and calorie counting by the middle class, further reinforced the trend toward lighter, simpler meals that had begun during the early 1900s. One-dish dinners, once despised as reflective of European immigrant peasant dishes, became very popular, as housewives discovered how much time and effort such dishes saved.

The "core" eating pattern. During this time, the foundations were laid for the meal plans that still persist as the core eating pattern of contemporary America. This general pattern includes breakfasts of citrus fruit or juice and dried cereal or eggs and toast, a light lunch of a sandwich, soup, or salad, and a dinner consisting of meat as a central entree with potato and vegetable side dishes, and a simple dessert (Levenstein 1988).

The use of canned goods continued to increase, particularly by the middle class. Jell-O, which had first found its way into American dining rooms in 1897 (General Foods Corporation 1962), became a popular, versatile food. Costing only pennies per package, Jell-O added welcome color and flavor to many an otherwise drab meal during the Depression. Mixed with canned fruits, it served as an attractive dessert. Along with mayonnaise and canned fruit or vegetables, it became widely used in making quick and easy salads, either for a main course or a side dish.

For those who could afford it, sliced baker's bread was a pleasant, convenient innovation. The ice-cream cone, which had come into being in

1904, was followed by the Good Humor Bar (with a stick) in 1920, and the Eskimo Pie in 1921. Popsicles appeared in 1924 (Root and de Rochemont 1976).

New restaurants. New kinds of restaurants developed to cater to the new lower-middle-class male and female office workers and shop employees who needed quick lunches at midday. During pre prohibition days, eating places (usually associated with bars) had been essentially male preserves. Now, restaurants became more attractive to women. Tea rooms flourished, attracting both women and men. Self-service cafeterias, (e.g., the Automats, which had been introduced prior to the 1920s) became big business when steam tables were added to provide the hot food then considered essential for a proper meal. By the mid–1920s cafeterias were beginning to give way to luncheon restaurants featuring even lighter foods. With the emergence of modified nutrition concepts (which came to full flower during the 1930s), the obsession with hot lunches faded, and sandwiches, salads, and other cold dishes became popular. Toasted bread, now conveniently prepared with the recently invented electric toaster, added a new dimension to sandwiches. "Luncheonettes" became popular. Drugstores also began to serve sandwiches and other food items at their soda fountains (American Restaurant Magazine 1932; Levenstein 1988; Van Leeuwarden 1920).

General trends. Many of the prudent eating habits engendered by Atwater's teachings of substituting cheaper foods for more expensive ones and general food conservation continued with renewed vigor, with the onset of the depression. Beans, peas, and cheaper cuts of meat were substituted for the more expensive meats. Thrifty homemakers used cooked cereals, rather than the more expensive commercial dry cereals. Although during the century from 1830 to 1930, pork consumption had decreased 25 percent from a yearly consumption of 178 to 133 pounds per capita, it still exceeded the consumption of beef, at 55 pounds per capita (Root and de Rochemont 1976; Burk 1961). Home gardens and home canning (Figure 6.8) played important roles in adding to the food supply during both the 1920s and the 1930s, as they did later, during World War II.

The role of home economists was strengthened, as they became increasingly linked to food industries. During this decade, diet kitchens became almost universal in the big food companies, manned by home economists. Some food companies developed a prototype home economist, or persona, to help promote their products. Perhaps the best known of these "home economists" is Betty Crocker of General Mills, Inc. She has survived the decades, providing consumers with helpful information regarding her company's food products (Figure 6.9). Supermarkets, many of them belonging to networks called chains, began operating throughout the United States during the 1930s. Their names (including Red Owl and Piggly Wiggly) became household words.

Consumption of alcohol. With the passage of prohibition laws effective

Figure 6.8
Peeling Apples for Canning, 1925

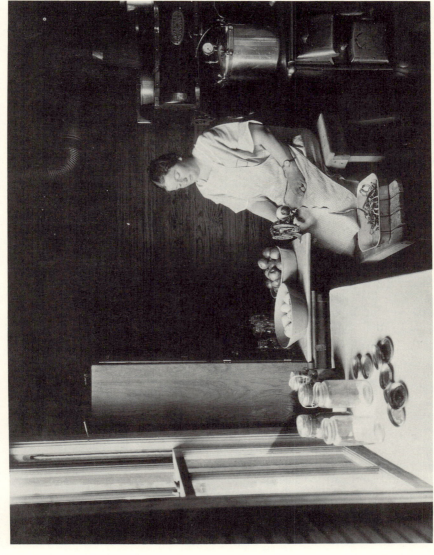

Photographed by G. Ackerman. United States Department of Agriculture (USDA).

Figure 6.9
Betty Crocker Has Survived the Decades

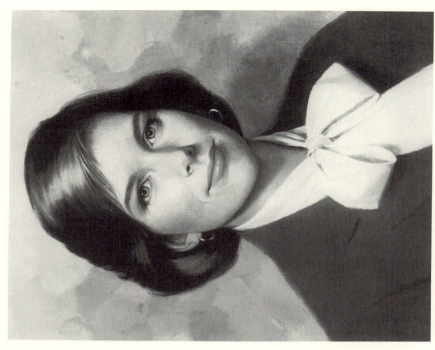

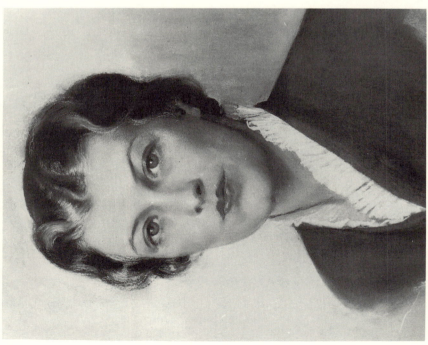

Left: as she appeared in 1936; right: as she has appeared since 1986. Used with the permission of General Mills, Inc.

115

January 14, 1920, the drinking of alcoholic beverages had decreased sharply. After repeal of the 18th Amendment in 1934, drinking increased again, particularly among the more prosperous.

Overview. That the Great Depression did not inflict more nutritional insult than it did, is undoubtedly due to the speed with which President Roosevelt's New Deal programs were put in place and their over-all effectiveness. The message of the nutritionists of the early 1900s and of Hoover's conservation program during World War I had fostered new habits and attitudes in Americans, which served as excellent preparation for the mandatory belt tightening that came as a result of the depression and drought. People had learned to get along (and surprisingly well) on less food and to make better food choices.

Many of the new attitudes and food patterns engendered by the Great Depression, coupled with expanded knowledge of nutrition produced a new focus, which emphasized good nutrition less as a means of treating diseases than for achieving optimum health. While Atwater's contributions had established the foundations for nutritional science, the subsequent discovery of vitamins and trace minerals revolutionized nutritional concepts, which were filtering down to the American public. By the time of the Great Depression the growing evidence that these nutrients were essential for growth, general health, and the prolongation of life had become widely accepted. Soon, research emphasis and ultimately public attention would shift toward the determination of the functions of these nutrients in human metabolism (Erdman 1989).

An interesting insight into the general "food picture" at the close of this era can be gained from the following description of food science in 1939:

Canning . . . [had become] a technology firmly under scientific control. By 1939, the use of refrigeration in the transport and the storage of perishable food became widespread, and frozen foods had begun to reach the retail level. There were roadblocks, however. Home refrigerators had replaced the ice box, but their freezers held only four ice cube trays. A popular venture capital business was installing neighborhood frozen food locker centers where you could conveniently keep your frozen foods only a few blocks away. Except for the recent and incomplete entry of frozen foods, there was no fresh seafood more than a hundred miles from the coast. Dried and salted (fish) was the rule. Lent was hell. Fresh oranges and lemons, apples, and vegetables were available fresh only when locally in season, and you enjoyed them when you could. (Hall 1989:188)

WARS AND RECOVERY, 1940–1960

As this period began, the Great Depression had not yet abated. Agriculture, which had been in an economic slump since 1920, was recovering from the Dust Bowl years. Yet within less than two years, the United States would become involved in a second world war. And as nations increased their production of war materials, providing jobs and putting larger sums of money back into circulation, the depression would end.

By 1940, food science had become strongly influenced by technology, with more than 65 percent of all food in trade channels passing through some stage of processing (Hampe & Wittenberg 1964). World War II served as a tremendous catalyst for the further development of food science (Goldblith 1989) and the food system in general. By 1940, nutritional scientists had succeeded in identifying, isolating, and characterizing virtually all of the essential nutrients. Now, their attention was shifting to determining the biochemical functions and mechanisms of action of those nutrients (Erdman 1989). Thus, the beginning of this period marked an important shift in food science toward food technology, as well as a major turning point for nutritional science.

By the end of World War II, of the major industrial powers, only the United States had been unharmed economically (Toffler 1980). The Korean war (between June 25, 1950, and July 27, 1953), in which the United States was heavily involved, effected a slight boost to the economy, with no overt effects on America's food system.

Food-related Developments

World War II and the food system. World War II had far-reaching effects on the American food system. The need to provide an adequate, safe food supply with optimum nutrition to the armed forces resulted in food rationing, as well as stimulating much government-sponsored research into new and improved food technologies and the setting of dietary standards. Fortunately, the entire American public benefited from these efforts, as did the total war effort.

Sugar, fats, meats and canned fruits and vegetables were rationed. As in World War I, these retrictions indirectly encouraged the increased consumption of eggs, milk products, and fresh fruits by civilians.

Research done by the Quartermaster Corps (Department of Defense) aimed at developing foods useful to fighting men under a variety of conditions resulted in improved methods of processing food, from which all Americans benefited. Much work was done on dehydration techniques, since dehydrated foods do not require refrigeration, are lighter (up to 99 percent of the water can be removed), and are easier to transport.

In 1940, the Food and Nutrition Board (FNB) of the National Research Council (NRC) was established to advise the federal government on nutrition as it related to national defense. Charged by President Roosevelt with the task of developing a set of dietary standards, to serve as a goal for good nutrition, the FNB developed the first set of Recommended Dietary Allowances (RDAs) within a year. Since this first edition (NRC 1943), pe-

Figure 6.10
Kitchen of New Pennsylvania Home, 1941

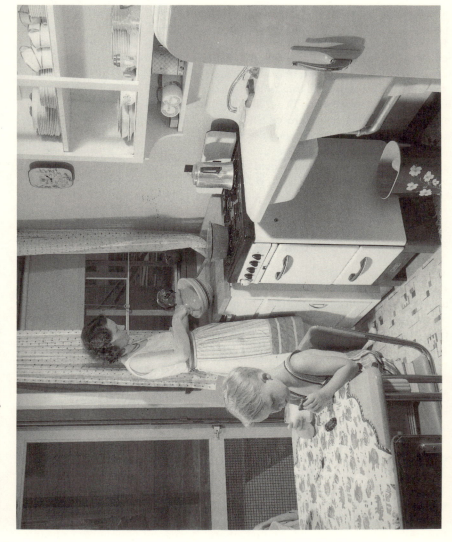

riodic revisions of the RDAs have been made, reflecting new scientific knowledge and interpretations. The most recent edition was published in late 1989 (NRC 1989). These standards represent recommended levels of intake for most healthy males and females of various ages with respect to energy (at differing activity levels) and those nutrients for which sufficient information is available to warrant making a judgment.

The enrichment of baker's bread (with thiamine, riboflavin, niacin, iron, and calcium) became mandatory in January 1943, until wartime legislation ended in October 1946. This legislation resulted from concern that certain vitamins and minerals were being lost during the removal of cereal hulls during the milling and refining steps of processing. Currently, although enrichment of foods in not required by federal law, more than half of the states require the enrichment of flours and breads. Since those companies wishing to engage in interstate commerce must enrich their cereal products, in practice, most of the flours, breads, and cereals on the market today are enriched. All enriched products now must be enriched with specified amounts of thiamine, riboflavin, and iron and must be appropriately labeled accordingly.

During the war years, it was required that oleomargarine be fortified with vitamin A and that milk be fortified with vitamin D.

Postwar advances in food processing. Although the use of frozen foods had begun in the 1930s, after World War II they become important competitors of other preserved foods available to consumers. Clarence Birdseye stands out as the pioneer most responsible for the creating of the frozen food industry. However, the scientific aspects of its development, which made frozen foods possible, were due to the efforts of men such as Dr. C. R. Fellers at the Massachusetts State College and Dr. Donald K. Tressler at Cornell University (Desrosier 1963).

The use of frozen, precooked foods began in the late 1940s, but increased tremendously during the 1950s with the introduction of the home food freezer (independent of the refrigerator). The complete meal (commonly known as the TV dinner) became a popular item in supermarkets by the mid-1950s, as well as frozen, ready-to-eat bakery goods.

Research on dried foods (much of which had initiated in response to the increased food needs of World War II) culminated in a number of food products that became commercially available. After 30 years of research, powdered (instant) skim milk came on the market in 1954. This product was prepared using the "agglomeration process" (Peebles 1958). Considerable quantities of orange and grapefruit powders, produced by the dehydration of fruit juices under high vacuum, were being sold by 1958. By this time, better technology also had improved the quality of dried eggs. Dried "instant" mashed potatoes were widely available by the mid-1950s. Both freeze-drying and air-drying were used for such products as coffee, tea, meat, fish, fruits and vegetables (Boggs and Rasmussen 1959).

By the end of the 1950s and the beginning of the 1960s, a large volume and variety of dried fruits (produced by sun-drying or mechanical dehydration) were being sold. The amount of dried vegetables on the market was relatively small, and limited in variety. Potatoes were the largest single item (Desrosier 1963).

Food packaging. The discovery of polyethylene and applications of polyvinyl chloride in the late 1930s, coupled with World War II, its food and material shortages, and the search for substitutes, led to widespread advances in food packaging during this era (Downes 1989). In addition to the more traditional wax paper and aluminum foil, housewives now were enjoying the use of such flexible, transparent products as Saran to cover their freshly prepared foods, as well as leftovers, before placing them in the refrigerator.

Fast food. The fast-food industry began in the 1940s, when White Castle, one of the first fast-food chains, opened its doors. Local carhop restaurants emerged, typically featuring root beer and other soft drinks, hamburgers, hot dogs, and French fries. These eateries included A & W Root Beer places and the fabulously successful drive-in restaurant in San Bernardino, California, known as McDonald's—run by Richard (Dick) McDonald. In the early fifties, McDonald and his brother, Maurice (Mac), introduced the Golden Arches concept and began selling McDonald franchises. Soon after, Burger King and Kentucky Fried Chicken also opened as fast-food restaurants (Bolaffi and Lulay 1989; Graham 1991).

Food safety. Important legislation, aimed at further safeguarding the food supply, was passed during the 1940–60 period. The Poultry Inspection Act of 1957 regulates all poultry and poultry products which enter interstate commerce. The Food Additives Amendment of the Federal Food Drug and Cosmetic Act of 1938 was enacted in 1958. It pertains both to intentional and incidental additives. This amendment contains the well-known Delaney Clause, also called the "cancer clause." The Delaney Clause states that "no additive shall be deemed safe if it is found to induce cancer when ingested by man or animal, or if it is found after tests which are appropriate for the evaluation of the safety of food additives, to induce cancer in man or animal." The Food Additives Amendment was the first legislation to prohibit the marketing of any additive until the Food and Drug Administration (FDA), after a careful review of test data, pronounced it safe at the intended levels of use. Data pertaining to safety must include toxicity tests on two or more species of animals. Additives already in use at that time, because of years of widespread use without harmful effects, were "generally recognized as safe" (GRAS) and exempted from this requirement. However, in 1977, the U.S. government directed the FDA to reevaluate all of the substances on the GRAS list (approximately 600 items). This tremendous task remains in progress.

School Lunch Act. In 1946, school lunch programs were expanded and

Table 6.1
Food Guides

Food Guide	Food Groups
Basic Seven[1]	Green and yellow vegetables Citrus fruit, tomatoes, raw cabbage Potatoes, other vegetables, fruits Milk and milk products Meat, poultry, fish, eggs, dried legumes Bread, flour, cereals Butter and fortified margarine
Basic Four[2]	Milk Meat Vegetable, fruit Bread, cereal
Six Food Group Pattern[3]	Breads, cereals, other grain products Fruits Vegetables Meat, poultry, fish, and alternates Milk, cheese, yogurt Fats, sweets, alcoholic beverages

[1]USDA 1943.
[2]USDA/ARS 1958.
[3]USDA/HNIS 1989.

strengthened by the School Lunch Act. The School Lunch program in the United States traditionally has had a markedly positive effect on the nutrition of school children, particularly the economically disadvantaged.

Dietary Guides

The year 1940 had ushered in a new era for nutritional science, which still is continuing—involving research into the biochemical functions and metabolism of essential nutrients. Federal agencies began to translate the new knowledge gained from research into practical dietary guidelines for consumers.

Eating guides. Home economists and nutritionists of the USDA developed a "7-Group Plan" during wartime, in 1943 (USDA 1943). Based on the RDAs published that same year, it was widely promoted as an eating guide (Table 6.1). A simplified version of the 7-group plan was developed, based on the RDAs of 1958 (USDA/ARS 1958). Known as the 4-group plan (milk, meat, vegetable-fruit, and cereal), it served for many years as the standard guide for nutrition educators and consumers with respect to food choices (Senauer, Asp and Kinsey 1991:52). It was influential in developing the concept of the "balanced meal" (i.e., that, ideally, a meal should contain foods from each of the four food groups). Both of these plans represented a core diet, with specified minimum servings from the food groups involved, determined by the age of the consumer. Additional calories, when needed, were to be supplied by additional servings from the designated foods groups or by fats and sugars. The latter could be consumed as such in miscellaneous foods such as baked goods and desserts. In 1989, a six-food plan was developed by the Health and Nutrition Information Service (HNIS) of the USDA (Table 6.1). This plan added a group for fats, sweets, and alcohol to the basic four, divided fruits and vegetables into separate groups, and added new foods to previous groups (USDA, HNIS 1989).

Eating Patterns, 1940–1960

During World War II the American public generally enjoyed an adequate diet, despite food rationing. Home gardens played an important role in augmenting the food supply during the war years of the 1940s. By contrast, the 1955 Food Consumption Survey (USDA 1957) showed that there was an abundance of food and that farm families were producing less of their own food than previously. A stimulated economy following World War II, plus new technologies, had dramatically changed the food system. Improved transportation, preservation, processing, and packaging produced a sharp increase in the numbers and types of food products available, and consumers were able to buy them. Norge Jerome (1981:41) says of this period, "No longer was diet variation limited to the physical environment, the season, or unsophisticated technology."

While grocery stores in 1916 had offered only about 600 items (American Dietetic Association 1988), supermarkets now carried several thousand items. Despite the dramatic increase in numbers and types of food products available within each food category, the actual foods consumed remained pretty much the same as in previous periods. The general eating patterns were the same as those developed during the 1920–40 period. Animal meat was considered an essential part of a meal, providing the focus for homemakers in planning their menus. Augmenting the meat entree were items chosen from a wide selection of foods: fruits, potatoes and other vegetables, grain products, dairy products, desserts and pastries. Energy expenditure had decreased because of the increase in sedentary occupations associated with urbanization, increased use of household appliances, the automobile, and other conveyances. The public's implicit attitude seemed to be that, if a certain level of nutrient consumption (e.g., protein) was good, more would certainly be better. This attitude was encouraged, at least in part, by the media.

THE SECOND AGRICULTURAL REVOLUTION, 1960–1980

By 1960, industrialism had peaked in the United States, and a postindustrial era was emerging (Toffler 1980). Within this context, agriculture was dramatically impacted, resulting in what is referred to here as the Second Agricultural Revolution.

Important Developments

Agricultural change. Agriculture entered a new era. The Rural Electrification Administration (REA) established during Roosevelt's presidency in 1935, had helped expand rural electric power development, so that, by 1960, more than 97 percent of U.S. farms had electricity. The use of commercial fertilizer increased dramatically, as well as the use of insecticides and herbicides (Figure 6.11). Improvements in farm equipment (Figure 6.12) and in livestock and poultry breeding, along with better nutrition and veterinary health care of farm animals, all led to higher farm productivity. Dramatic advances in crop breeding also occurred. By the early 1960s, more than 95 percent of all U.S. corn acreage was planted with hybrid seed (Figure 6.13). The result was a sharp increase in overall agricultural production. During this period, each farmer was producing enough food for more than 70 people. Less than 3 percent of Americans were now living on farms, most of which were owned by individuals.

The beginning of this period saw the initiation of serious efforts on the part of developed countries to improve agriculture in poor countries. During the 1960s, scientists introduced varieties of wheat and rice that gave much higher yields than earlier varieties. These new varieties were especially helpful to poor countries, who desperately needed increased crop yields to feed their burgeoning populations. Various agencies of the federal government (such as the Department of State's Agency for International Development and agencies within the Department of Agriculture, together with international agencies such as the United Nations' Food and Agriculture Organization (FAO) and the World Bank, have made invaluable contributions toward the improvement of agriculture in the Third World. This collective effort often has been referred to as the Green Revolution.

Nutrition and poverty. The decade of the 1960s was influenced strongly by the presidential terms of two Democrats, John F. Kennedy (1961–63) and Lyndon Johnson (1963–69), characterized by Kennedy's New Frontier Program and Johnson's Great Society. Americans had become increasingly aware that the economic rebound following World War II had not erased poverty completely in the United States. A U.S. Senate Subcommittee on Employment, Manpower and Poverty started an investigation on the problems of hunger in April 1967. Their observations during visits to Mississippi and other target areas were dramatically presented in a televised

Figure 6.11
Weed Control Through Herbicides

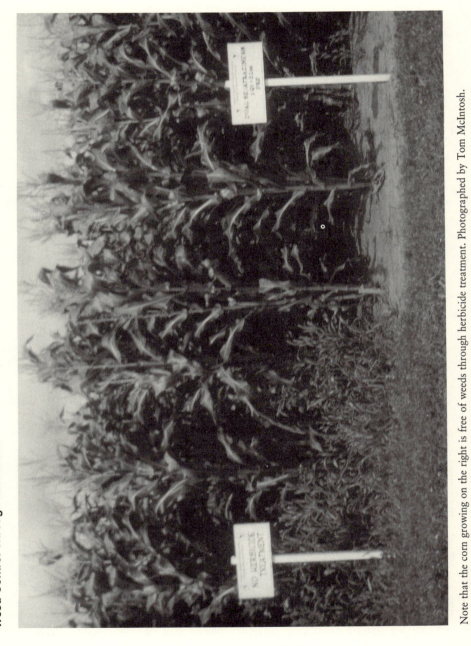

Note that the corn growing on the right is free of weeds through herbicide treatment. Photographed by Tom McIntosh.

Figure 6.12
Harvesting Wheat with Combine

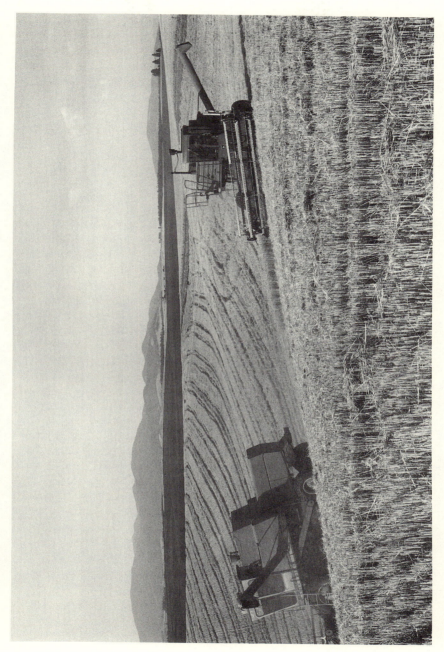

Agricultural Research Service, USDA

Figure 6.13
Hybrid Vigor Resulting from Crossing Two Inbred Corn Strains

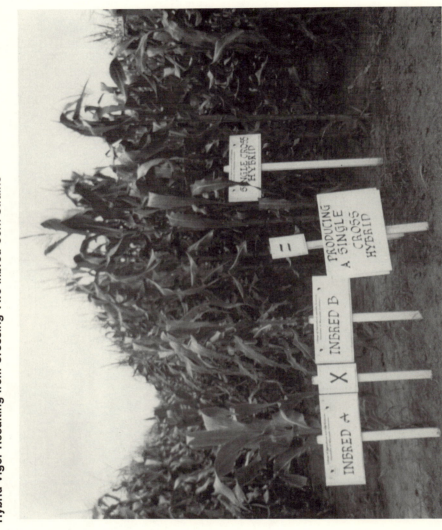

Note the dramatic increase in plant height and vigor in the single cross hybrid (right). Photographed by Tom McIntosh.

feature program in April 1969 called "Hunger in America" (Columbia Broadcasting System 1969). These and other activities served to increase public awareness of the problems of hunger and poverty and to create a climate of concern which extended into the 1970s.

The War on Poverty (part of Johnson's program) was formally launched by the passage of the Economic Opportunity Act of 1964. "It included initiation or expansion of a wide variety of programs designed to provide the poor with a safety net of basic income, medical care, food and shelter, or as with job training, and educational programs, to offer an escape from poverty" (O'Hare 1985:10). Important legislative actions included the Food Stamp Act of 1964 and authorization for the Headstart program in 1965. Because of the many community nutrition and other social programs that proliferated during this period, this decade often had been referred to as the Glorious Sixties.

The 1970s were characterized by a continuation of the public interest in nutrition that had developed during the 1960s. In 1972, Congress passed legislation authorizing the Special Supplemental Food Program for Women, Infants and Children, often called WIC (Special Supplemental Food Program 1975). This program is funded and administered by USDA through state health departments and Native American tribes, bands or groups. In 1974, the Food Stamp Program became a nationwide program operating throughout the United States and territories based on a uniform set of federal rules (USDA 1976). Two major nutrition programs designed especially for the elderly, the Congregate Meals Program and the Home Delivered Meals Program were authorized by legislation in 1972 as an amendment to the Older Americans Act of 1965. All persons who are over age 60 are eligible to receive meals from one of these programs, regardless of their income level. By the late 1970s, reduced federal funding began to force cutbacks in certain nutrition-related programs and to curtail efforts to launch new ones.

Food-related Developments

General trends. By 1960, the food industry had grown at a rate faster than the general economy (Hampe and Wittenberg 1964). The 1960s saw dramatic growth in successful home food delivery in the United States. This enterprise had begun in the late 1950s with home-delivered pizza, followed by other menu items (e.g., Chinese food). During the 1970s, Wendy's popularized drive-through windows (Bolaffi and Lulay 1989). Diet foods became available during the 1960s; during the 1970s, "health" and "organic" foods became available, especially in specialty shops. By the 1970s, "healthy" foods were evolving as a major staple in food service operations (Bolaffi and Lulay 1989). By 1978, 10 percent of the households in the United States owned a microwave oven.

Figure 6.14
Sealing Jars of Canned Goods Using Two-Piece Metal Lids, 1975

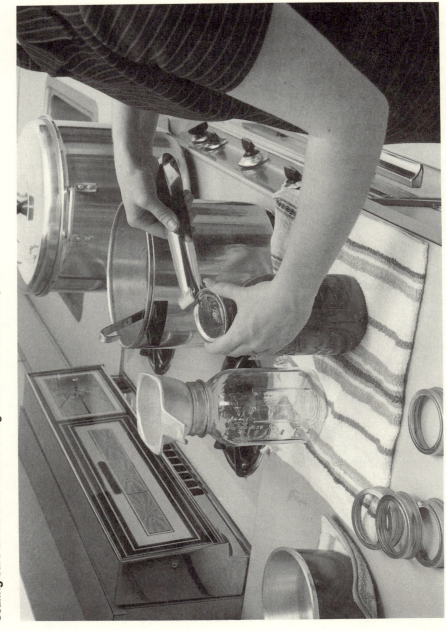

Photographed by Fred Faurot. United States Department of Agriculture (USDA).

Food packaging. Important milestones in food packaging during this period included the development of plastic tubs for cottage cheese (1960), high-density polyethylene (HDPE) gallon milk jugs (1961), all-aluminum beer cans and polyethylene-coated milk cartons (1962), easy-open aluminum ends for beer cans (1964), screw-off closures for beer bottles (1965), laminated plastic tubes (1965), plastic-foam egg cartons, clear PVC bottles for food (1968), large bottles for soft drinks (1970), "bag-in-box" for wine (1976), and polyester soft-drink bottles (1977). The aseptic carton was introduced in the United States during the 1980s (Sacharow and Brody 1987; Lund 1989). Essentially a paper bottle, it is used in aseptic processing whereby shelf-stable food products are produced by sterilizing the product and its container separately, then filling the container with the product in a sterile atmosphere (Downes 1989). This technique provides increased food quality and retention of nutrients.

Food safety. In 1966, the Congress authorized the FDA (of the U.S. Department of Health, Education, and Welfare [USDHEW]), to set up requirements for complete information in labeling and for packaging that is not deceptive with respect to its content. The Fair Packaging and Labeling Act went into effect July 1, 1975. The law defined the layout of the label. Labeling is required for any food to which a nutrient has been added or for which a claim is made regarding nutritional value (USDHEW, FDA 1975).

Eating Patterns of the Period

Changing food tastes. Food was abundant, both in quantity and diversity, encouraging overindulgence in food. For those who could afford it, a trend toward "dietary individualism" developed (Jerome 1972; 1979), engendered in part by a tendency toward increased assertion of self.

Although for most Americans, meat continued to occupy a central place in the meal, with other foods playing a subordinate role, alternative dietary patterns were developing. For a variety of reasons, many people began to question the traditional American emphasis on food, and especially the consumption of meat. Plant foods began to occupy an increasingly important place in the diet, with a deemphasis of animal meats, especially beef.

Increased demand for plant foods was coming not only from native-born Americans, but also from immigrants, most of whom were now arriving from Southeast Asia, Latin America, or the Caribbean—areas whose meals traditionally have emphasized multiple vegetable dishes (Jerome 1981). Many Americans became vegetarians, of one type or another. Others professed a preference for so-called natural foods.

Increased racial pride led to the revival and increased visibility of traditional southern African-American cuisine, which came to be called soul food in the 1960s (Kittler and Sucher 1989). Many ethnic groups also demonstrated increased interest in their native cuisines during the 1960s and 1970s.

The food system responded accordingly to these changes in food preferences by making more of the desired foods available. The result has been even greater possibilities for variety in the American diet.

These changes were shaped, in part, by the social climate of the 1960s, with a widespread questioning of the status quo, American involvement in Vietnam, and deep concern for the environment, including pollution and foods safety. Many activists questioned the wisdom of using food additives, for whatever purpose. Members of the new generation, born into an era of technology, with its plastic, "ersatz", artificial, man-made concoctions, had a deep yearning to go "back to basics." This desire often translated to acquiring an acreage in the country and producing one's own food. In contrast, many members of the older generation, who had grown up on farms, had experienced, firsthand, the drudgery associated with food production (e.g., cleaning a steamy, stenchful henhouse or endlessly weeding a garden). They recognized and appreciated the advantages that this era of technology now offered.

Diet and health. During this period, there was a subtle turning away from the implicit, if not overtly articulated ideology of the 1950s that "more is better" as far as food and nutrition was concerned. After a long hiatus, the public was rediscovering the nutrition adages preached by Atwater and his nutrition colleagues at the turn of the century. By the late 1970s, the evidence was mounting that the lowering of blood lipids in the human diet was associated with reduction of plaque size (and hence, regression of atherosclerosis) (Blankenhorn 1978; Gotto 1979).

Food, health, and poverty. Added to the prevailing mood of the 1960s was the growing evidence that, indeed, there were things wrong with the nutrition of many Americans. Health professionals, particularly nutritionists and physicians, were becoming increasingly concerned over the high prevalence of diet-related chronic diseases and conditions. In addition, there was public concern over hunger and malnutrition, particularly among the poor, in the United States. These concerns were being widely discussed in the media. The diverse pressures that rose from this climate of concern ultimately led to the establishment of the Senate Select Committee on Nutrition and Human Needs in 1968 and the White House Conference held in 1969.

Dietary goals. Perhaps more than any other factor, the hearings carried on by the Senate Select Committee led to the increased sensitivity and awareness of diet and health in the United States (Senate Select Committee 1968). One salient outcome was the establishing of dietary goals and guidelines (Senate Select Committee on Nutrition and Human Needs 1977). Table 6.2 shows the third edition of the dietary guidelines (USDA and USDHHS 1990). These dietary recommendations are extremely relevant to

Table 6.2
Dietary Guidelines for Americans

1. Eat a variety of foods.
2. Maintain healthy weight.
3. Choose a diet low in fat, saturated fat, and cholesterol.
4. Choose a diet with plenty of vegetables, fruits, and grain products.
5. Use sugars only in moderation.
6. Use salt and sodium only in moderation.
7. If you drink alcoholic beverages, do so in moderation.

Source: USDA/USDHHS 1990.

the prevention of such chronic health conditions as obesity, hypertension, coronary heart disease, cancer, and diabetes (Type II). With the publication of these recommendations, the preventive nutrition era began in earnest (Erdman 1989).

THE BIOTECHNOLOGICAL REVOLUTION (1980–PRESENT)

This period has been characterized by postindustrialism. Alvin Toffler (1980:10) has described this era as "at one and the same time, highly technological and anti-industrial." Modern biotechnology has made giant strides forward (see next section and chapter 10). This period also has been distinguished by efforts toward "wholism," by diversity, and by alternative lifestyles. Collectively, these influences are effecting significant changes in American living, including food habits.

Food-Related Developments

Biotechnology and new food products. Broadly defined, biotechnology involves the use of living organisms or processes to make or modify products, to improve plants or animals (Figures 6.15 and 6.16), or to develop microorganisms for specific uses (U.S. Congress, Office of Technology Assessment 1992). Biotechnology is not new to the agriculture and food sectors. Living systems have been used for thousands of years for the production of foods. Well-known examples are bread, cheese, sausage, and alcoholic beverages. However, "the modern era of technology began in 1973, when scientists cut a gene (a small piece of DNA) out of a cell from Xenopus and spliced it into a tiny bacterial chromosome (plasmid). The ability to specifically cut and recombine genes led to the development of what is now known as recombinant DNA technology" (Etherton 1992:13). The terms "biotechnology" and "genetic engineering" should not be used interchangeably, since the former encompasses a vast array of techniques

Figure 6.15
Genetic Engineering of Plants

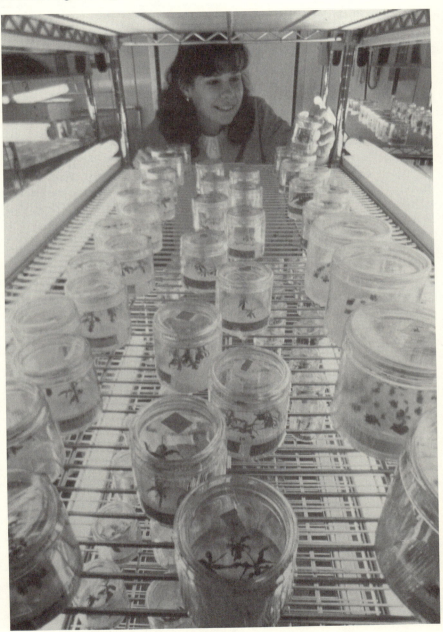

Scientist checks on tiny peach and apple trees produced through genetic engineering. Agricultural Research Service, USDA.

Figure 6.16
Genetic Engineering of Animals

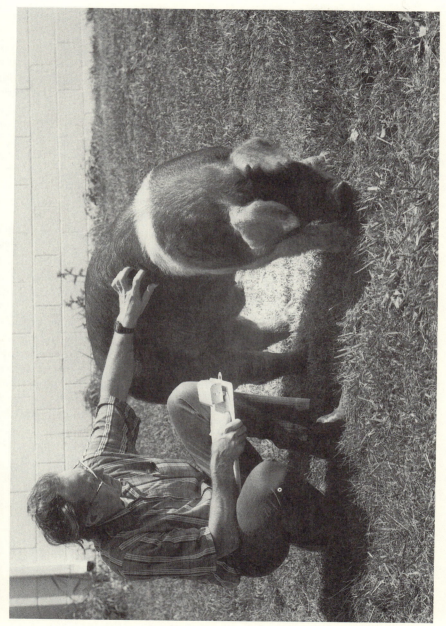

Animal physiologist examines pig whose embryo was implanted with a bovine growth hormone gene through genetic engineering. Agricultural Research Service, USDA.

and processes, only one of which is the splicing of genes (genetic engineering).

The first impact of biotechnology on the food system has been in production agriculture, that is, improvements in the yield of plant products at the farm level. These improvements are being effected through the development of disease-resistant, herbicide-tolerant, and insect- or virus-resistant plant varieties by selection in tissue culture or by genetic engineering techniques. These same technologies have been used to develop salt-tolerant, temperature-tolerant, or drought-resistant crop varieties (Harlander 1989). Biotechnology has a tremendous potential for impact on agriculture and the food system in the near future (chapter 10).

Abundance of foods. At present, continuous advances in food science and technology combined with the demands of an increasingly heterogeneous American society are resulting in an unprecedented selection of foods available to the American public. Supermarkets today carry 24,000 items (American Dietetic Association 1988).

Microwave ovens. Today, at least three out of four households in the United States have microwaves. By the year 2000, it is projected that 90 percent of American households will have one. Food processors are developing new products and adapting existing ones to meet the present and anticipated future demands for microwavable foods (Institute of Food Technologists 1989).

Fat substitutes. In response to the desire of consumers for foods lower in fat content, the food industry has developed several low-calorie and calorie-free fat replacements and fat substitutes. Most of the ingredients being promoted as partial or complete replacements for fat belong to one of three major categories: protein-based substitutes, synthetic compounds, and carbohydrate replacements (Kirkegaard 1989). The use or potential use of any food substitute depends on the food product, replacement level, and initial fat content.

Protein-based fat substitutes are low-calorie ingredients derived from protein found in eggs, milk, and other foods. Simplesse, which belongs in this category, was introduced in January 1988 by the Nutrasweet Company, Skokie, Illinois. The first product made with Simplesse was a frozen dairy dessert called Simple Pleasures, introduced by Nutrasweet in February 1990 (Institute of Food Technologists [IFT] 1990).

Synthetic compounds used as fat substitutes are fatlike substances that are resistant to hydrolysis by digestive enzymes as partial or complete replacements for fats and oils. Olestra is the proposed generic name for sucrose polyester (SPE), a nonabsorbable synthetic fat produced by the Proctor and Gamble Company, Cincinnati, Ohio. This product currently is undergoing review by the FDA (IFT 1990).

For over a decade, some carbohydrates and carbohydrate-based materials have been used to replace fats and oils (partially or totally) in a wide variety of food products. These products include gums, polydextrose (produced by Pfizer Chemical Division, New York), Corn Starch Maltodextrin (Maltrin M040, produced by Grain Processing Corporation, Muscatine, Iowa) and others (IFT 1990). In KRAFT FREE Nonfat Mayonnaise Dressing, introduced by Kraft General Foods in 1990, cellulose gel is used as a fat replacement (Freedman and Gibson 1991).

Sweeteners. Along with calorie-containing sweeteners, consumption of artificial sweeteners has increased. The two newest artificial sweeteners (approved by the FDA) are aspartame and acesulfame-K. Aspartame (commonly known by the brand name Nutrasweet) has been widely available since the early 1980s. About 200 times sweeter than sugar, it is approved for use in a number of products. Equal is the only brand of tabletop sweetener that contains aspartame. Acesulfame-K, introduced in 1990, is also 200 times sweeter than sugar. It is marketed as Sunett and as an ingredient in Sweet One, a granulated product used like sugar. Ace-K has the advantage of retaining its sweetness in baking; however, it does not produce the same texture in baked goods as does sugar (Mayo Foundation for Medical Education and Research 1990).

Nutrition Labeling and Education Act. The nutrition label, which until recently, was provided on many food products, was developed in the early 1970s. At that time, the predominant focus of public nutrition was on micronutrients. Since then, consumer awareness and interest in diet/disease relationships has risen dramatically (Levy and Heimbach 1990), and the focus of public nutrition has shifted to macronutrients. The Nutrition Labeling and Education Act of 1990 (Public Law 101-535), which went into effect in March 1994, represents a response to the public's changing nutritional concerns. A major premise of this act is that it should assist consumers in maintaining healthy dietary practices. Using the information now provided by the new labels, consumers should be able to reduce consumption of total and saturated fat, increase fiber intake, and (if necessary), reduce calorie intake (Wallingford 1994).

Diet and health. The focus on preventive nutrition, which began in the late 1970s, gained momentum during the 1980s. Based on the Dietary Goals published by the Senate Select Committee in 1977, the USDA and USDHHS jointly issued the first edition of the Dietary Guidelines in 1980 (USDA/USDHHS 1980). (The third edition of these guidelines [USDA/USDHHS 1990] is shown in Table 6.2.) In 1982, the National Cancer Institute published an initial report containing related guidelines for reducing cancer risks. These guidelines echo those of the Dietary Guidelines with respect to dietary intakes of fat, fiber, and alcohol. In addition, they urge consumers to limit use of food preserved by salt curing (including salt pickling), smoking, or nitrite curing (National Cancer Institute 1982). Subsequent reports have been consistent with these initial recommendations.

Since these two sets of guidelines were released, their message has permeated the thinking of the American public.

Since 1980, there has been an overwhelming emphasis on diet and health, both in the areas of nutrition research and in its applications to American food habits. The importance of diet for overall health promotion and disease prevention has been brought to the attention of the public by the government, the food industry, and by innumerable professional and consumer groups, as well as the mass media (Erdman 1989; Monsen 1989).

The 1980s were years of tremendous growth in the prominence of nutrition and dietetics. The word "nutrition" was launched into the headlines more than in any previous decade (Monsen 1989; O'Neill 1990). These trends have continued during the 1990s.

Eating Patterns of the Period

Current trends. Societal changes are influencing how, where, and when people eat (American Dietetic Association 1988). Perhaps the most profound change is the increased number of households that consist of two working parents, a single parent, or all working adults. As a result of these changes in family structure and lifestyle, there are increasing trends toward more meals eaten in restaurants, more foods eaten at home which have been prepared elsewhere, and a greater use of convenience items in foods prepared at home.

In addition, there has been a trend toward the replacement of the traditional three meals per day with "ad hoc" meals (American Dietetic Association 1988). The consumer is demanding a greater variety of "heat and eat" foods. Along with fast food, the use of take-out and home delivery of foods is increasing. The observation that the United States has become a nation of snackers and grazers is frequently made.

Fast foods. The fast food phenomenon, which took off in earnest in the 1950s, has since grown into a multibillion dollar business that now accounts for 40 percent of the money spent on meals away from home by consumers. In 1987, the three leading fast-food chains were McDonald's, Burger King, and Kentucky Fried Chicken, with annual sales of $14.1, $5.6 and $3.7 billion, respectively (Shields and Young 1990).

The popularity of fast food stems from many factors: reduced time for food preparation, with more women in the work force; a greater number of people who live alone and lack the incentive to cook for themselves; less formal lifestyles; convenience of fast-food restaurants; increased amount of disposable income; and increased opportunities for recreation and travel. Additionally, there is increased awareness of fast foods due to extensive advertising, and Americans simply like fast foods, and the prices are relatively reasonable (Shields and Young 1990).

Because so many people are consuming fast food, both health professionals and consumers are concerned about its nutritional quality. Meals from fast-food establishments tend to provide adequate amounts of carbohydrate and B-complex vitamins. However, they have been criticized for their generally high calorie, sodium, fat, and cholesterol content. These meals also tend to be low in calcium, dietary fiber, and vitamin C.

During recent years, the fast-food industry has responded to these criticisms. They have expanded their offerings to include such foods as grilled chicken sandwiches, breakfast items, baked potatoes, chili, and fresh and packaged salads. Additionally, in 1986, at least five of the major chains decreased their use of saturated fat, switching from an animal-vegetable shortening to an all-vegetable product for all-purpose frying (with the exception of French fries). This change heralded a continuing trend toward reduced use of saturated fat in the preparation of fast food. Health professionals are hopeful that the fast-food industry will be able to reduce total fat content as well, as fat substitutes become more available.

Snack foods. The market for snack foods is growing by more than 10 percent each year. People are buying more soft drinks, chips, crackers, and cookies.

Ethnic foods. Ethnic foods exploded into the mainstream of the American diet and food service establishments during the 1980s (Bolaffi and Lulay 1989), a trend which continues.

Nouvelle cuisine. A new trend in cooking emerged quietly in the early 1970s in France, when Paul Bocuse, along with other young French chefs, began to develop a new, "minimalist" style of cooking. It was a counteraction to the stuffiness of French haute cuisine of the early years of the century. Food critics hailed the early efforts of these chefs as the beginning of a worldwide revolution in taste. The new dishes were served, not with the traditional flour-thickened sauces, but in reduced stocks from the natural juices of cooked meat. There was a new emphasis on fresh ingredients (with their intrinsic tastes retained), al dente vegetables, raw fish and meat, and a new interest in rediscovering regional cooking (Sokolov 1991:223–38). In a new concern with visual effects, food tended to be served on very large plates, with studied placements of julienned (sliced) vegetables, arranged in circular or other geometric patterns. By 1980, French nouvelle cuisine restaurants had opened up in the United States on both coasts. Since then, this cooking style has insinuated itself into the cuisine of upper-scale restaurants throughout America.

Two-tiered approach to cooking. Many busy homemakers have found that there simply is not time to prepare gourmet dinners every night of the week. They are solving this problem by serving fast food or meals that are already at least partially prepared but indulging in more time-consuming meals when time permits (e.g., weekends).

Consumption of alcohol. Although sales of beer and wine have increased greatly since 1949, alcohol consumption, generally, has dropped significantly (see chapter 10).

FOR FURTHER READING

Douglas, P. 1930. *Real wages in the United States, 1890–1926*. Boston: Houghton Mifflin.

Etherton, T. 1993. The new bio-tech foods. *Food and Nutrition News* 465(3):13–15.

Goldblith, S.A. 1989. Fifty years of progress in food science and technology: from art based on experience to technology based on science. *Food Technology* 43(9):88–107, 286.

Hampe, E.C., and M. Wittenberg. 1964. *The lifeline of America—development of the food industry*. New York: McGraw-Hill.

Levenstein, H.A. 1988. *Revolution at the table*. New York: Oxford University Press.

Root, W., and R. de Rochemont. 1976. *Eating in America*. New York: Ecco Press.

Senate Select Committee on Nutrition and Human Needs. 1977. *Dietary goals for the United States* (2nd ed.). December. Washington: USGPO.

Senauer, B., E. Asp, and J. Kinsey. 1991. *Food trends and the changing consumer*. St. Paul, MN: Eagan Press.

Steinbeck, J. 1939. *The grapes of wrath*. New York: Viking Press.

Toffler, A. 1980. *The third wave*. New York: William Morrow and Company.

USDA/USDHHS. 1990. *Nutrition and your health: Dietary guidelines for Americans* (3rd ed.). Home Garden Bull. 232. Washington: USGPO.

7

Understanding Food Habits

Throughout history, food has had special meaning and significance for humankind. Those people who did not eat well tended to die. Thus, humans became aware that food is of the utmost importance for everyone, in order to survive. Because food fulfills basic physiological needs essential for life, food soon took on special social and psychological significance. Food is something with which every living person has had contact, usually on a daily basis, throughout life, or that individual would not have survived. Therefore, all of us have had an intimate familiarity with food, perhaps making us feel qualified to evaluate and discuss issues which surround it. For all of these reasons, there are few topics which elicit more emotional responses and on which people have stronger opinions, than food.

All societies have, throughout time, shared the same intense interest and reverence for food. And, historically, they have possessed similar, predictable appetites for certain types of foods. These appetites are largely physiologically and genetically based. Yet, the specific foods that different groups or individuals actually choose from the environment to satisfy these needs may vary widely from group to group, or even among individuals within a group. Different groups may have completely different attitudes toward a given food. For example, grasshoppers are considered a rare delicacy in certain Middle Eastern societies; most Americans cringe at the thought of eating this insect. Americans will eat only eggs which are fresh

Figure 7.1
Family Picnic at Park, c. 1948

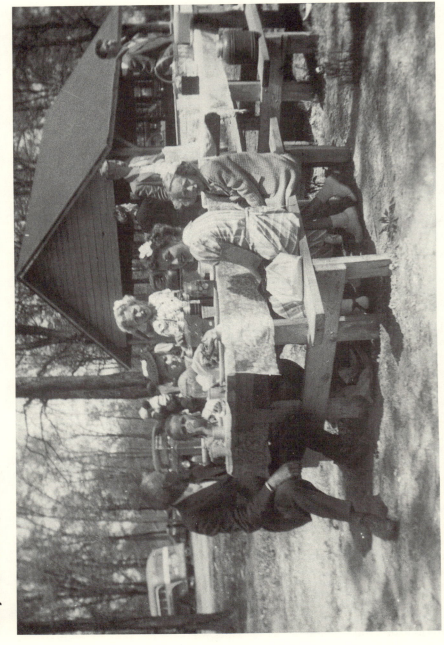

and infertile; an egg containing a partially developed chick embryo is considered to be a delicious food in China.

Over time, certain groups of people build attitudes for and against certain foods. They are most likely to approve of familiar foods that have proven, over time, to be nontoxic and conducive to optimum health and performance. Thus, a body of attitudes eventually develops with respect to foods that are potentially available in the environment of the group.

Individuals within a group (and youngsters, especially), as a result of various subtle conditioning methods (e.g., approval from the group when making certain choices, disapproval when making others), slowly take on the food habits of the group. This standardized body of food behaviors become the food habits of the group. Originally serving to guide members of the group toward making ideal food choices, the sharing of common food habits ultimately becomes a mechanism for expressing group identity and/or maintaining group boundaries.

Thus, like most aspects of culture, food habits develop as a collection of eating behaviors that have proven to be most advantageous to the group's members. Over time, these accepted behaviors become a blueprint for optimizing the chances of survival both for individuals and the collective group.

Nao Wenkam stated that

Eating is learned behavior. We're born without a system of eating habits but are reared so that, as adults, we become hungry at certain times for particular things, with definite attitudes toward food; we adopt a nutritional behavior pattern which we refer to as food habits. (Wenkam 1969:1)

FACTORS AFFECTING FOOD CHOICES

A close look at dietary patterns shows that they are affected by interactions among many factors, which can be categorized broadly as biological, environmental, and cultural. Within these categories are numerous subfactors. A listing of these factors (not necessarily inclusive) is presented in Table 7.1.

To be successful, a diet first must meet a human individual's minimal nutritional needs, so that people within a cultural group can live and reproduce. Otherwise, that society will not survive. The foods in the diet must contain sufficient energy and essential nutrients in a physiologically available form. In other words, the body must be able to digest, absorb, and metabolize the ingested foods.

Beyond the basic biological need for sufficient energy and nutrients from food that is physiologically available, environmental factors become the most crucial determinant of dietary patterns, since a food can be used only

Table 7.1
Factors Affecting Food Choices

Biological Factors
    Nutritional needs
    Heredity
    Special physiological conditions (e.g., pregnancy)
    Special diseases or abnormal conditions
    Taste preferences (genetically determined)
    Individual cravings or idiosyncracies

Environmental Factors
    Geography, climate
    Season
    Economics
    Transportation
    Technology
    Fuel availability

Cultural Factors
    Education
    Understanding of nutrition/health concepts
    Income
    Social class, status
    Traditions, beliefs, values
    Ideology (worldview, religion)
    Communication
    Influence of business, government, professionals
    Politics

if it is available. Many factors influence environmental availability (Table 7.1).

In addition to biological and environmental availability, and as Table 7.1 shows, food choices depend on many cultural factors. To begin with, different groups, and even individuals within that group, despite having similar items present in their environment, may have differing attitudes as to which ones are acceptable as food. In addition, there are diverse ideas regarding given foods, as to how they should be obtained, prepared, and consumed. Ultimately, cultural factors determine which of those items in the environment that are physiologically utilizable will actually be chosen for consumption and under what conditions.

In addition to these three broad categories of factors (and their sub-groups) (Table 7.1), food habits can be influenced by complex interactions between categories and/or subgroups. For example, physical status may affect the cultural availability of a food. By way of illustration, in certain primitive cultures a woman or child may have limited access to meat. Most cultures have both dietary prescriptions and proscriptions (taboos) for women during pregnancy. Within certain groups in Hawaii, pregnant women are warned against eating double or multiply joined bananas to ward off multiple births or joined digits (Wenkam 1969). All of us have heard the old wives' tale that strawberries may cause a birthmark on the developing fetus. Many cultures forbid pregnant women to eat fish, for fear that the newborn may be born with scaly skin.

Biological Factors

The prime biological need is for adequate nutrition, which includes effective digestion, absorption, and metabolism of ingested food. Thus, wise food choices are essential to life. Early man had to learn by trial and error which foods were edible. The ability to select those foods which are nutritious and reject those which are poisonous obviously conferred a survival advantage. All humans today possess certain genetically determined predispositions that promote adaptive food choices (Rozin 1987; see section on taste preferences in this chapter).

Heredity also can influence food choices. For example, adverse reactions to certain foods sometimes have a genetic basis. The inability to tolerate cows' milk may be caused by a reaction to foreign proteins (a heritable predisposition) or to lactase deficiency (which can be either a heritable or an acquired trait). Diabetes mellitus (the inability to utilize glucose normally) is a common metabolic disorder with a strong heritable basis.

There are many special diseases or abnormal conditions (both hereditary and nonhereditary) which influence or restrict food choices, and nutritional needs strongly affect food choices and are affected by several factors. They include gender, age, and special physiological conditions.

Male babies are born with less mature nervous and digestive systems than female babies. Thus, they are more likely to be colicky and less efficient in processing food than girls. Because males have a higher basal metabolism rate than females, they tend to have higher energy needs than females of comparable size, age, and physical activity.

Age affects food choices across the life span. During infancy and childhood, the need for nutrients is high, to support growth. Considering their great need for nutrients, babies are at a distinct disadvantage with respect to their ability to utilize food. They are born without teeth, with poor swallowing ability, and with digestive capabilities which are not completely developed. Hence, a baby's first food must be liquid, nutrient dense, and easily digested. Fortunately, these criteria are met by breast milk and most infant formulas. As the young human grows and matures, the ability to utilize food increases, along with the range of feasible food choices. As a person ages, digestive, absorptive and metabolic capacities decrease, along with chewing and swallowing capacities, so that food choices again become progressively restricted.

Pregnancy affects food choices in several ways. During the early months, nausea and vomiting often restrict food choices to bland, well-tolerated foods. After three months, basal metabolism increases, along with appetite. There is an increased need for energy and most nutrients. These factors all translate to increased food intake. Nutrition education for the pregnant woman is very important, so that this increased intake will consist of wise food choices; the diet should provide those nutrients which are essential to both the mother and developing fetus. The diet of the pregnant woman should consist of foods high in protein, minerals (especially calcium and iron), and vitamins (especially vitamin C and the B vitamins).

The pregnant woman frequently has individual cravings. While the cause of these cravings is not fully understood, they frequently are attributed to the increased basal metabolism and increased nutrient needs, particularly during the last two trimesters of pregnancy. Highly individual food cravings and preferences are not confined to pregnant women (see sections on taste preferences, unique food combinations, and pica in this chapter).

Environmental Factors

The physical availability of foods is a powerful determinant of food choices, since one cannot eat what is not available. Geography and climate have closely associated effects on food availability, because they influence which foods are grown in a given area. Most people tend to eat more of those foods which are locally produced, particularly when they are in season. Season of the year affects food choices since foods are more available in season and at cheaper prices. In Third World countries, where good transportation and commercial infrastructures are marginal, foods tend to be consumed with a one-half-mile radius of where they are grown. As a result, at harvest time, there often are more fruits and vegetables available than can be consumed readily. Thus, considerable food goes to waste. In more developed areas, various food preservations techniques (e.g., refrigeration, freezing, canning, and drying) allow storage in situ or make it possible to ship these surplus food products to distant places outside the immediate area. Fuel availability is an important factor in food choice, because some foods tend to be unsuitable for consumption unless cooked; cooking also helps to preserve foods.

Adequate distribution of food is dependent on a number of factors. In addition to availability of transportation and food-processing techniques, food distribution is influenced by economic conditions and political factors.

Cultural Factors

Cultural factors (Table 7.1) affect food choices in diverse, subtle, and all-encompassing ways. Whether a food that is physiologically and environmentally available actually is consumed depends on a culture's attitude toward that food. Attitudes toward food, in turn, evolve from a society's traditions, beliefs, and values, and strongly influence individual food behaviors.

Each individual belongs to a number of groups. In addition to the larger society, an individual belongs to several successively smaller units. Of all group influences, the prime influence seems to be the family (Cussler and deGive 1952; May 1957) (Figure 7.1), though friends and shared interests have their own effects (Figure 7.2).

Parents exert an undeniably strong influence on the eating patterns of their offspring. Initially, they have complete control over what foods are offered the baby. And their control remains strong during childhood, since parents determine which foods come into the household.

A baby is born with a strong instinct to put all materials indiscriminately into its mouth, a survival behavior which helps insure that sufficient nourishment will be obtained. A baby beginning to crawl and explore the environment uses newly developed pincer skills to pick up diverse small objects, in addition to food. Even items such as dead flies, matchsticks, and debris may be taken into the mouth. Such behavior typically galvanizes parents into action. Using various intervention methods, accompanied by expressions of approval or disapproval (as appropriate), parents ultimately teach their toddler to differentiate between what constitutes food and what does not (McIntosh 1987). Moreover, youngsters slowly begin to like those foods which are served often. These foods invariably include staples, which take on high significance and meaning through repeated exposure.

Education and understanding of nutrition/health concepts are important factors in influencing food behaviors, because they enable individuals to make informed food choices. Social class and status also shape food habits, since many foods are categorized as appropriate or inappropriate for a given social class. Food habits are also affected by ideology (worldview and religion) (see chapter 8). Religious precepts often dictate both prescriptions and proscriptions for certain foods. Income is important, because it determines the kinds and quantities of food that can be purchased. Political factors also play an essential role in determining access to food.

Communications and the influence of business, government, and health professionals on food patterns have become increasingly important, particularly in the industrialized countries. Politics also impact food habits because they can affect food availability.

The impact of communication(s) on food habits cannot be overestimated. Since the first gesturing by early humans to one another to indicate where food could be found, followed by halting vocal utterances and graphic representations of edible plants and animals in caves, people have been sending messages to their peers regarding food. From earliest times through the present, one of the strongest means of communication with respect to

Figure 7.2
Dining Room at Hidden Valley Resort, 1963

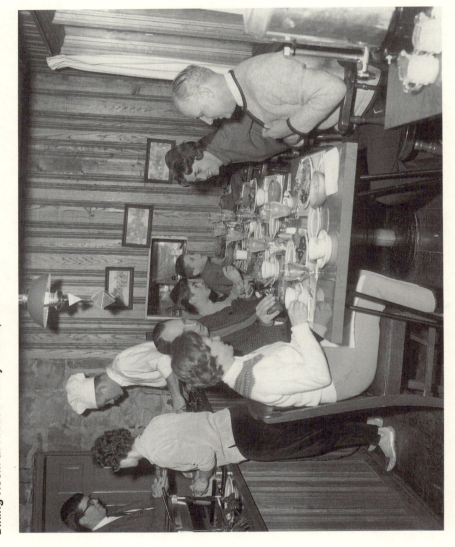

Photographed by Clarence Deland. United States Department of Agriculture (USDA).

food has been by observation—watching what people eat and how they prepare food. As civilization progressed, hand-produced cookbooks were developed and distributed (chapter 3). After the invention of the printing press came newspapers and magazines that advertised various foods and conveyed food information. Since the early 1920s, radio has been an additional, important medium for food communications. Finally, the introduction of television in the early 1950s has exerted a tremendous impact on food habits, including the acceptance of new foods. On television, viewers actually see people prepare exotic or ethnic foods, watch commercials for ethnic and "pop food" eating places, and observe celebrities endorsing diverse kinds of foods. It is interesting that, in addition to the ready availability of the above-mentioned sources of food information, more cookbooks are now being published, purchased, and read than ever before.

TO EAT OR NOT TO EAT?

Perceptions of Edibility

Early people had to learn by trial and error what foods were edible. The ability to select those foods which were nutritious and reject those which were poisonous obviously constituted a survival advantage. All humans today possess certain genetically determined predispositions that promote adaptive food choices (Rozin 1987).

The classification process that each individual uses to determine what is considered a food was well described by the Committee on Food Habits of the National Research Council (1945) and resummarized by Kittler & Sucher (1989:13):

1. Inedible foods: those foods which are poisonous or are not eaten because of strong aversions or taboos.

2. Edible by animals, but not by me: for example, foods such as insects in the United States or corn in France, where they are considered to be feed grains.

3. Edible by humans, but not by my kind: these are foods that are viewed as acceptable in some societies, but not in one's own culture. Examples of unacceptable foods in the United States which are acceptable elsewhere are dog meat in Asia and horse meat in Europe.

4. Edible by humans, but not by me: these foods include foods that are generally acceptable by a person's cultural group, but not by specific individuals, because of personal preferences or aversions, cost, health reasons, or other factors.

5. Edible by me: All those foods selected by the individual for his/her diet. These items may include certain highly individual foods or combinations (see section on Unique Food Combinations).

From the foregoing, it can be seen that perceptions of edibility exert a prime influence on food choices, because individuals understandably tend to eat only those foods which they consider to be edible. Certain foods considered edible in one culture may not be considered edible in others. As food becomes scarce, the criterion of edibility tends to become progressively relaxed, so that ordinarily forbidden foods such as animal or human feces, or even the flesh of one's own kind, may be consumed.

Taboos

As indicated above, the perception of edibility is heavily conditioned by the society in which one lives. In all cultures, concepts of edibility tend to become progressively relaxed as food becomes scarce, so that formerly forbidden foods may become condoned. "Choices are made only when food is plentiful enough to permit choices" (Lowenberg et al. 1979:103).

Cannibalism. The history of all societies (including our own) reveals that during starvation, its members have resorted to cannibalism. The prime example in the annals of American history is the tragedy of Donner Pass, which cuts through the Sierra Nevada mountain range in eastern California. During the severe winter of 1846–47, a party of settlers from Illinois and adjoining states became snowbound there. Running out of available food, many starved to death. Others resorted to eating the dead (Bartlett 1989).

Food aversions. According to Rozin (1987), many, if not most, food aversions arise because of beliefs that ill health or misfortune may result from the consumption of various substances. He suggests that the term "taboo" should be reserved for those aversions which are backed up by religious views of obedience to the will of a deity. The need for the additional reinforcing effect of sacred interdictions against the eating of certain foods may arise from ambivalence and ambiguities regarding a food. Marvin Harris (1979:192–95, 248–53) noted that taboos are likely to arise when the systemic cost/benefits of an item shift from favorable to adverse, as a consequence of ecological and infrastructural changes. The topic of taboos is explored in greater depth in chapter 8.

TASTE PREFERENCES

Humans have innate, biologically based preferences for sweet and slightly salty substances and an aversion to sour and bitter ones. These preferences undoubtedly are based on physiological needs, while the inborn aversions may serve as a protective mechanism, since many poisonous substances taste bitter. The body seems to react to intense tastes of any kind (Lyman 1989).

Taste preference also can result from combined biological and cultural influences. While the ability to distinguish among sweet, salty, sour, and bitter tastes is shared by all societies, preferences for certain tastes vary greatly between cultural groups. For example, Mexicans like hot and spicy foods, such as chili peppers, which most Americans find too strong. Paul Rozin (1987:189–91) has described the liking of chili peppers as an acquired liking for an innately aversive food. Since chili peppers promote salivation, they undoubtedly aid in mastication of dry and mealy foods. They also may well improve the taste of the bland Meso-American staple— the tortilla. The ability of humans to convert an aversion to a liking is unique and include such favored substances as tobacco, coffee, the irritant spices, and the various forms of alcohol (Rozin 1982).

UNIQUE FOOD COMBINATIONS

Foods chosen by the individual may include food combinations not commonly accepted. These often may be snack combinations, originally chosen at random from what was available during a late night foraging expedition among the contents of the refrigerator. The combinations may have proven to be unexpectedly palatable and thus indulged in again. Often these preferences are carefully guarded, perhaps to avoid risk of censure from one's cohorts. Examples of unusual combinations (not highly publicized) are mayonnaise and peanut butter, jelly and pickles, chocolate cake with dill pickles, and pickles and peanut butter.

Some traditionally accepted combinations include roast pork and applesauce, strawberries and cream, apple pie and cheddar cheese, liver and bacon, fish and chips, pork and beans, and hamburgers and French fries.

PICA

People who have pica most frequently crave clay, laundry starch, or ice. However, eating such diverse materials as chalk, burned matches, coffee grounds, or even tire inner tubes also has been reported (Bryant et al. 1985).

Geophagia (clay eating) has been noted throughout history, worldwide. However, it is most common in tropical countries. In the United States, the highest incidence is among southern African Americans, whose clay (and dirt) eating often is engaged in surreptitiously. The secretive nature of this activity seems to stem less from fear of censure than from fear that others might discover the user's prized cache of clay.

What causes pica? Five major hypotheses have been proposed to explain this condition (Bryant et al. 1985):

1. It results from the body's need for certain nutrients.
2. It represents a mechanism for alleviating hunger.

3. It has a psychological or emotional basis.
4. It is a cultural phenomenon passed from generation to generation.
5. It is a response to physiological changes.

In evaluating pica practices and their possible etiology, Elaine McIntosh (1986) suggested that there may be a common motivational basis for pica, applicable across the sexes, among both the poor and the affluent. This underlying factor is deprivation, of one or more types, e.g., insufficient food, inadequate nutrients(s), lack of oral satisfaction, lack of external stimuli (e.g., boredom), or emotional deprivation.

Pica can have numerous undesirable effects on both nutritional and medical status (McIntosh 1986). Fortunately, most people who practice pica consume only modest amounts of foreign substances, so that complications are relatively rare. It is obvious that more research needs to be done on the phenomenon of pica. Pregnant women represent a particularly vulnerable group who should be monitored (adroitly and tactfully) by health care providers for potentially dangerous pica practices.

USES AND MEANINGS OF FOOD

Survival

Throughout history, the fundamental use of food has been to appease hunger and to provide nourishment for the body. Because food is so essential for survival, it has become imbued with a special significance that goes beyond that of satisfying hunger and bodily needs.

Progressive Uses of Food

Miriam Lowenberg et al. (1979) have used Abraham Maslow's hierarchy of human needs (1970) to explain the progressive uses of food from eating to satisfy hunger and bodily needs to using food as a means of self-actualization. Maslow classified human needs as physiological, safety, belonging and love, esteem, and self-actualization. These basic needs can be fulfilled in part by food.

Physiological (survival) needs. The physical need for food to satisfy hunger and provide nutrients is the most basic use of food. This need must be satisfied first before food can be perceived as a vehicle for satisfying further needs.

Safety (security) needs. Once short-term hunger needs have been met, people become interested in building up food supplies (or financial security) to ensure sufficient food for the future. People who are most motivated to can, freeze, or accrue large amounts of food supplies are frequently those who, earlier in their lives, have known episodes of having insufficient food.

Belonging and love. These needs are pursued next. Consuming those culturally familiar foods which tend to be used by the group gives an individual a sense of belonging. Sharing common diets is a means of expressing and maintaining ethnic identity and group boundaries. Although food habits are to a large extent evolutionary, they are maintained in part through deliberate means. People tend to eat together. Thus, eating common food together is another way in which food contributes to a feeling of belonging. (A bride and groom, sharing the first piece of wedding cake, is an example of the association between togetherness and food.) Often, food is used to express love and friendship. All societies use food as gifts. An example of food being used to express love: mothers typically prepare favorite foods for individual members of the family. While food can be used to express love, it can also serve as a substitute for love (e.g., too much chocolate cake, candy, rich sundaes).

Esteem (or status). The uses of food can enhance esteem or confer status upon an individual in two ways. First, the act of eating with someone denotes social equality with that person. People tend to eat with equals rather than those perceived to be above or below them in social status. In most societies, servants tend to eat by themselves in the kitchen, away from the family. Most societies have rules regarding who can dine together which serve to define and maintain class relationships. Second, foods themselves tend to enjoy individual status. Certain foods (usually scarce or expensive, and/or out of season, such as caviar or macadamia nuts) enjoy a relatively high status, while others, such as fat side pork and pork liver, are held in lower esteem. Certain brands of foods or beverages also enjoy higher status than others.

Self-actualization (or self-realization). This is the ultimate human need. Food can be used to satisfy this need by experimenting with special, creative recipes, special ingredients, gourmet cooking, and the preparation of special dinners with a unique ambiance (e.g., using fine linens, china, tableware, candlelight).

Obviously, food can fulfill several or all of these needs at the same time. For example, people may give lavish dinner parties as a means of deriving status, and also as a creative outlet.

For many individuals, not all these needs will be fulfilled. People who fail to achieve the most basic need for food starve to death. Many people throughout the world strive throughout life to fulfill only the most basic survival need of food. Still others are rarely able to build up food supplies or security beyond the present. Most of the world's people are content if food also fulfills needs for belonging and love. Relatively few people are in a position to use food as an expression of status. Food used as a means to achieve self-fulfillment, although relatively rare, has been observed among the affluent throughout history.

Other Uses and Meanings of Food

Another role of food is that it provides simple gustatory pleasure (Lee 1951). This is a complex feeling, resulting not only from a pleasing taste but also from the oral satisfactions of chewing and swallowing.

Some societies (e.g., the Quakers) regard eating as a duty or virtue, since the ingestion of food is essential for life. They also may value sameness and monotony in food (Lee 1951).

Emotional weights of meals and foods. The relative emotional weights of specific meals and of various foods are important considerations in effecting changes in food habits. In virtually all societies, the meal with the least emotional weight is the first meal of the day (breakfast), and the one least likely to be eaten with other members of the family. The meal with the most emotional weight universally seems to be the evening meal (dinner), which tends to be shared by all members of the family. Served at the end of the day, when the work of the family is done, and family members can relax, it tends to take on the focus of a family ritual. In some societies, the meal, consisting of several courses, and interspersed with visiting, storytelling, and drinking of alcoholic beverages, may continue for several hours.

Special status of staple foods. Foods also have varying emotional weights. The foods most frequently eaten are called staples or core foods (Passim and Bennett 1943). In many societies, one food is so basic that its members feel they cannot live without it. They develop a reverential regard for this food (Mead 1955). In many Asian cultures, the staple is rice, which is considered to be an essential component of every meal. For Hispanic Americans, foods made from corn (e.g., tortillas) and beans are staples. In the United States as in Ireland, potatoes have been a staple. Wheat was the staple of early agriculturists in the Holy Land; its hallowed status is reflected in the many biblical references to wheat and bread, as well as symbolic uses of the word bread (e.g., "bread of life").

Significance of salt. When early man became an agriculturist, the relatively low amount of sodium in the plant foods predominately eaten, plus the constant loss of sodium through perspiration in the warm climates where early man was concentrated, created a need for salt sources extraneous to the amount found in the early agriculturist's regular diet. Thus, salt assumed a position of great importance and symbolism. Because salt is so essential to survival, human settlements often were chosen which were close to a source of salt (first obtained by evaporating sea water, and later, by mining it from naturally occurring deposits). Wars have been fought over salt. The importance of salt is reflected in the Bible in such passages as Matthew 5:13: "You are the salt of the earth."

Emotional release. The role of food as a means of relieving tension is well known. The physical act of eating and drinking, plus the rise in blood sugar associated with eating, promotes a feeling of well-being and satiety. While most people tend to nibble more under stress, others tend to eat less.

Symbolic meanings of food. Sweet foods are often used as a substitute for love and a feeling of comfort. Consumption of sweet foods often increases during times of tension.

Milk is associated with deep feelings of love and security, for several reasons. First, it is the initial food ingested by infants, in association with a warm breast or nippled bottle. Then there are the oral satisfaction of suckling and the emotional comfort of being cradled in the arms of a significant other. American travelers and servicepeople alike, after being in foreign countries, have reported that safe and pasteurized milk was the food they most missed.

MEALS, MEAL PATTERNS, AND MEAL SERVICE

The analysis of eating patterns serves as a valuable method of defining food habits (Douglas 1972). Important characteristics of meal patterns within a culture include what constitutes a meal, the accepted elements of a meal, the order in which these elements are served, how many meals are eaten per day, and when. Other significant aspects include which foods are appropriate for a given meal (e.g., breakfast), who prepares the meal, how it is prepared and served, who eats the meal, and with whom. In addition, periodic fasting or feasting (or both) frequently are meaningful components of the meal cycle (Kittler and Sucher 1989). Fasting (either complete or partial) customarily is associated with a religious observance. Feasting always celebrates a significant event: a religious or secular holiday or a personal rite of passage, such as birth, marriage, graduation, or death. Fasting and feasting are discussed further in chapter 8. Thus, the study of meals and meal patterns shows that food and how it is used conveys powerful messages about social relations, important religious and personal events, and many other aspects of a culture.

Meals

In all cultures, a meal consists of a main course and side-dishes. In the United States, a formal meal begins with appetizers, followed by soup or salad, then the main course, and finally, dessert and coffee. A family meal follows this same general order; however, not all of the elements may be included. Because of calorie consciousness, Americans now frequently omit bread and desserts. The main course (or entree) consists of meat, chicken, or fish, potato or pasta, and a vegetable.

People in poor countries may eat only one meal per day. However, in more affluent societies, three or four meals are traditional.

In all societies, eating together (usually with people perceived as equals) is a symbol of liking and trust. Thus, dinners usually are reserved for family and friends. In the United States, business associates and acquaintances tend to be invited for cocktails and hors d'oeuvres, which often are consumed while standing. The latter practice dismays many foreign visitors, who sometimes avow they simply "cannot eat standing up".

Meal Patterns

In the United States, three meals have been considered traditional, served in the morning, at noon, and in the evening. When the country was primarily rural, the timing of meals was determined by the daily demands of farm work. Breakfast was a hearty meal, consisting of cooked cereal, bacon (or steak), eggs, toast, milk and coffee. The midday meal, called dinner, was the largest, designed to meet the energy needs of the afternoon's activities. The last meal of the day, somewhat lighter than the noon meal, called "supper," was served after the field work was done. With increasing industrialization, people migrated to towns and cities, where meals began to conform to factory and business schedules. Breakfast became a much lighter meal, and its time depended on the individual urbanite's work schedule. The midday lunch was usually consumed at the factory, during a short break. Often brought from home, it was much lighter than the midday meal served on the farm and became known as "lunch." For a factory worker, it made more sense for the largest meal of the day to be served in the evening, and it became known as "dinner." At least until World War II, whether a person referred to meals as breakfast, dinner and supper, or as breakfast, lunch, and dinner, quickly identified the individual as being of rural or urban origin. More recently, the words "lunch" and "dinner" for the midday and evening meals may reflect a higher status. And the word "supper" may describe a special late meal (usually of the upper class), such as at midnight at New Year's, post-theater, or on Sunday nights.

Three meals a day is still traditional in the United States. However, a survey in the mid-1980s revealed that only two out of five Americans eat the traditional "three squares" a day. About 25 percent admitted that they frequently skip either breakfast or lunch on a given day. Nutritionists agree that the meal most likely to be skipped, by adults and youngsters alike, is breakfast.

In other societies, there often are more than three meals a day, some of which are little more than a beverage and/or small snack. In the Scandinavian countries, there may be as many as six meals of various sizes per day. The first is a very light meal of coffee and possibly a pastry served in one's room, followed by "breakfast" later in the morning, served in the dining room. In England, the four o'clock tea with biscuits (cookies) has been a tradition, followed by dinner at about seven in the evening. In tropical countries, shops may close around midday for several hours, while people go home, eat, and take a nap during the heat of the day. They then come back to work later in the afternoon, working on into the evening. The hour for dinner thus may be nine o'clock or later, at least for the adults.

Meal Service

While it is customary for foods to be served at a table in Western societies, most of the people of the world eat on the floor, as has been done historically. Globally, most people still eat with their fingers, often from a common pot (another universal practice). A contemporary example is the serving of poi in Hawaii at luaus. Two fingers are dipped into a bowl containing a sticky mass of poi and then returned to the bowl for a second helping. Visitors are often repelled by this practice, in part because of the danger of spreading disease.

Tableware is a comparatively recent phenomenon. The first eating utensils were undoubtedly made of wood (such as spoons and chopsticks, still used today). By the Middle Ages, most Europeans carried an all-purpose knife, which they also used for cutting meat and bread. However, fingers still were the customary eating tools. Small forks were used at table in Byzantium as early as the tenth century. From Byzantium, their use spread progressively to Greece, Italy, and France (in 1533, when Catherine de Medici went to France to marry the dauphin). Later, they were introduced to England. However, most Europeans continued to eat with their fingers until the eighteenth century, when the dinner fork finally became commonly used (Tannahill 1973).

In early colonial America, most of the settlers made their own tableware of wood (e.g., spoons and trenchers). However, wealthy colonists imported household articles (including tableware) from England. Later, colonial craft workers began making many household items, including table utensils, from silver and pewter. Silverware became more and more common, particularly after the Revolutionary War, in the urban cities of the Eastern seaboard (Tannahill 1973; Martin 1989a).

Individual dishes also are a relatively new arrival to the dining scene. Historically, and even today, many of the world's people prepare foods in such a way that individual dishes are not absolutely essential. In many cultures (e.g., in the Middle East), breads constitute an essential component of the meal. Flat breads, especially, are used as a plate or receptacle for holding other food. Pita bread (with a pocket for holding chopped meats, cheese, and vegetables) is another example of a meal that requires no plate. In medieval times, pies, pastries, and fritters consisting of meat, sauce, and a plate in one self-contained package, were commonly served. In addition, each individual carried his own trencher, a thick slice of stale unleavened bread about 6 by 4 inches, which acted as an absorbent plate. In about the fifteenth century, the bread trencher began to be replaced by a square of wood with a round depression in the middle, used both in Europe and in the Colonies. More affluent persons began to use pewter trenchers (Tannahill 1973).

Many early cultures began making useful household utensils from baked clays as early as 6000 B.C. Collectively called pottery, these wares are classified as earthenware, stoneware, or porcelain, depending on the mixture of clays used and the temperature at which the pottery is fired. Most of the tableware used in Western societies today are representative examples of these three types of pottery.

Pottery-making spread from Egypt and the Near East to southern Europe. The first pottery undoubtedly was earthenware. Techniques for making stoneware spread to Europe from China, where it was first produced during the fifth century A.D. Porcelain products ("china") first made by the Chinese during the Tang dynasty (A.D. 618–907), were brought by traders to Europe as early as the 1100s. By the 1700s, porcelain manufactured in Europe was competing with Chinese porcelain (Gates 1989). Thus, techniques for making these three types of dinnerware were well known in Europe by the time American colonization began. While most settlers used wooden trenchers for a plate, the more affluent colonists imported pottery from England. Soon, the settlers began making their own earthenware and stoneware. However, because the Europeans guarded their secrets for making porcelain so carefully, china continued to be imported. Today, excellent brands of U.S. porcelain are available.

STABILITY OF DIETARY PATTERNS

Two old sayings are that "given a choice, man tends to eat what his ancestors ate before him" and that "man tends to prefer those foods that he's used to." These adages still hold true. Children slowly learn to like foods that are frequently served. In fact, it is common knowledge that young children usually prefer the same foods day after day. Some groups regard sameness and monotony in food to be a virtue (Lee 1951).

Immigrants cling more tenaciously to eating habits than to clothing and language after their arrival in the United States. One reason for this behavior is that food confers identity, and this can be done privately in the home, free from possible censure by indigenous Americans (outsiders). Immigrant women, in general, are slowest to adapt to new ways. Early immigrant women, especially, tended to be cloistered in the home, slower to learn English, and more likely to follow traditional customs.

The elderly, as a group, are also resistant to change. They, too, cling to their customary eating habits, regarding change as threatening (particularly when they are not feeling well, as under typical hospital conditions).

Traditional eating habits are being challenged as never before by many influences. Young and middle-aged American adults tend to prize variety in their diets. They are constantly exposed to the influences of business and the media, which tout the many new food products made possible by advanced food technologies. The latter are bringing a host of new flavors, textures, and characteristics to well-known foods.

APPROACHES TO UNDERSTANDING FOODWAYS

The study of food habits makes it obvious that they are influenced by physiological, environmental, and cultural factors. Of these, cultural factors are in many ways the most difficult to define, because they are so diverse and pervasive, varying from culture to culture.

Anthropologists tend to use two theoretical approaches in examining foodways. The etic approach, which is more common, involves data collection and observations made by persons outside the culture. The emic approach involves eliciting the viewpoint of persons within the culture. Attempts are made to ascertain "the participants' sense of what people eat or ought to eat, and the symbolic significance of food preferences and avoidances" (Harris 1987).

Most of us nurture tenacious biases regarding food habits, which reflect our own cultural conditioning and experience. For this reason, anthropologists who wish to understand another culture typically live intimately within that cultural group for an extended period of time, to help gain an insider's perspective.

Certain food habits within a culture that at first glance may appear repugnant, unwise, or without basis to an outsider have probably evolved over time for complex, compelling, adaptive reasons. Often, professionals from outside the culture, assuming that their foodways are superior, will seek to replace indigenous food patterns with ones more like their own. This ethnocentric approach can sometimes have disastrous results.

In evaluating food habits, ethnocentrism must be avoided as much as possible. Instead, professionals must "learn to suspend judgment, to strive to understand what goes on from the point of view of the people being studied" (Hoebel and Frost 1976:23). Ideally, one should approach new situations, including foodways and people, with an open mind.

FOR FURTHER READING

Bryant, C.A., A. Courtney, B.A. Markesbery, and K.M. DeWalt. 1985. *The cultural feast*. St. Paul, MN: West Publishing Co.

Cussler, M., and M. deGive. 1952. *Twixt the cup and the lip*. New York: Twayne.

Harris, M. 1987. Foodways: historical overview and theoretical prolegomenon. In M. Harris and E.B. Ross (eds.), *Food and evolution* (57–90). Philadelphia: Temple University Press.

Kittler, P.G., and K. Sucher. 1989. *Food and culture in America*. New York: Van Nostrand Reinhold.

Lowenberg, M.E., E.N. Todhunter, E.D. Wilson, J.R. Savage, and J.L. Lubawski. 1979. *Food and people* (3rd ed.). New York: John Wiley and Sons.

Lyman, B. 1989. *A psychology of food*. New York: Van Nostrand Reinhold.

Mead, M. 1955. *Cultural patterns and technical change: a manual prepared by the World Federation for Mental Health*. New York: New American Library.

Rozin, P. 1987. Psychobiological perspectives on food preferences and avoidances. In M. Harris and E.B. Ross (eds.), *Food and evolution* (181–205). Philadelphia: Temple University Press.

Tannahill, R. 1973. *Food in history*. New York: Stein and Day.

Wenkam, N.S. 1969. Cultural determinants of nutritional behavior. *Nutrition Program News*. July/August.

8

Food and Ideology

Society has several functions. In addition to reproduction, socialization, the production and distribution of goods and services, and the preservation of order, a prime function is the maintenance of a sense of purpose.

Historically, people have looked to ideology to fulfill this basic need for a sense of purpose—involving the conviction of a supreme being who controls the destiny of all. Ideology encompasses a society's beliefs, meanings, and values, which tend to be expressed symbolically through mythology and religion, folklore, dance, literature, and language. It includes all of a society's concepts about the world and man's place in it. Even a society's food habits reflect its ideology. Three related aspects of ideology which exert special influences on dietary patterns are worldview, mythology and religion, and health beliefs. This chapter will focus on the influence of myths, religious beliefs, and associated rituals on the food practices of followers of the world's major religions.

RELIGION, MYTHOLOGY, AND RITUALS

Religion

Religion is a system of beliefs expressed through rituals and other practices through which man relates to a supreme being and whereby human life attains meaning. Historians of religion believe that some form of relig-

Figure 8.1
The Seder Table

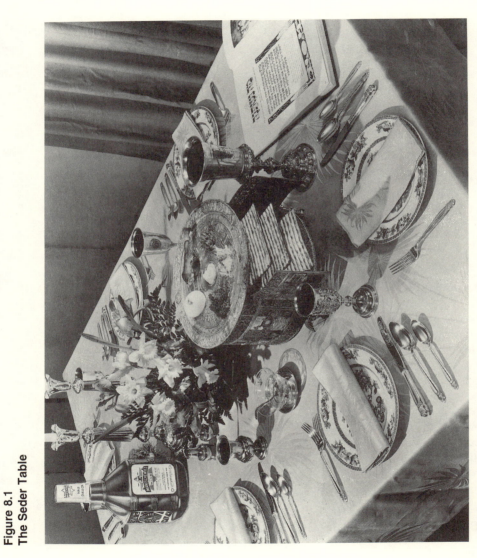

Table set up for Passover, showing Seder plate containing matzo and other symbolic foods. Courtesy of the B. Manischewitz Company, Jersey City, N.J.

ion has been practiced since the first human beings evolved some 1.5 million years ago. These early people were confronted by many things they could not understand. It is thought that very soon they developed the belief that spirits lived in and controlled all things in nature. People began to worship these spirits because they were so powerful. Scholars believe that religion originated out of this worship.

Mythology

These early societies developed stories through which they tried to describe how the spirits or sacred powers directly influenced the world. These stories, called myths, usually involved deities or demigods and showed how some natural event in the world was indirectly caused by the supreme beings. Historically, in unrelated cultures the world over, many myths have described the creation of the world, or how the human race or a particular people began. Other myths provided explanations for the cause of natural occurrences such as thunderstorms or the changes of the seasons. Thus, myths, which are an integral part of religion, have helped people make sense of unexplainable happenings and have served to allay anxiety regarding the unknown. The religious significance of myths separates them from folktales and legends, which are told primarily for amusement.

Religious Rituals

Myths have played an important part in each society's religious life. Religious leaders often used these stories to dramatize the teachings of their faith, by incorporating them into religious rituals. A religious ritual essentially is an enactment of a myth. Jack Campbell (1988) believed that a religion began when an enlightened leader translated some of his visions into ritual performances for his people.

Each religion has evolved certain rituals or customs that are important to the members of that religion. The observance of these rituals is believed to be mandatory since they express and reaffirm the various beliefs of the religion. Myth and ritual have played a tremendous role in the religious life of numerous societies, beautiful pictorial examples of which are shown by Oliver La Farge (1956).

RELIGION AND FOOD

Prehistoric people centered their religious activities on the most important elements of their existence, such as the prosperity of their tribes and getting enough food to survive. These early people performed religious ceremonies to ensure a sufficient food supply. People in hunting cultures drew pictures and performed dances to ensure good hunting. Later, agriculturists performed ceremonies at planting time to help ensure a good harvest. They also made sacrifices, for the same reasons. Early people often placed food, ornaments, and tools in graves, believing that these items would be useful to, or desired by, dead people.

Thus, many religious rituals and practices involve food. Many proscriptions and prescriptions regarding food have their origins in mythology, which are part of the belief systems of selected religions. The various religions of the world have had a profound influence on man's dietary practices and customs. Over the centuries, religions often have decreed what foods humans could or could not eat, what foods they could or could not eat on certain days of the year, and frequently, how certain food must be prepared for consumption. Many of these dietary habits have become symbolic of the religion itself. In fact, regulations regarding food and drink serve as the glue that promotes the cohesion of members of a given religion. For a long time, anthropologists have recognized the role of food in religion, especially as related to taboos, feasting, fasting, and sacrifice.

Why this interrelationship between religion and food? Since food was early man's most essential (and often scarcest) possession, it is understandable that it became associated with many of his religious rituals or customs. For example, the giving of food, or abstaining from food, to secure the goodwill and protection of the all-powerful being (or beings) has been common since primitive times. In the attempt to appease these deities, early humans often offered them their most precious possession, food—the best that they had. The practice of fasting evolved from attempting to gain approval from the gods by abstaining from food.

The idea of sacrifice (including food) also stems from the desire for appeasement, or approval, with respect to the gods. Historically, guilt and sacrifice have been integral components of both Judaism and Christianity. An example of sacrifice is the case of Abraham offering up his eldest son, Isaac. To Christians, the death of Christ on the cross symbolizes the ultimate sacrifice (atonement for the sins of humankind), which is central to Christian ideology. These well-known examples represent attempts to gain approval, appeasement, or atonement from a supreme being.

THE FIVE MAJOR RELIGIONS: INFLUENCES ON FOOD HABITS

Christianity

An outgrowth of Judaism, Christianity began in A.D. 30, when Jesus was crucified in Jerusalem. His followers spread Christianity to major cities throughout the Roman Empire, and, ultimately, throughout the world. Today, Christianity constitutes the largest religious group in the world, with about 1.7 billion followers. Most Christians are members of one of three major groups: Roman Catholic (56 percent), Protestant (20 percent), or Eastern Orthodox (9 percent). Christianity has had an enormous influence on Western civilization.

Roman Catholics. Traditionally, Catholics were required to observe certain fast days and to refrain from eating meat on Fridays in remembrance of Christ's sacrificial crucifixion. However, the United States Catholic Conference abolished this ruling in 1966. Catholics now need abstain from eating meat only on Fridays during Lent.

Protestants. Most Protestant denominations show little involvement of food as part of their religious beliefs and observances, with the exception of their sacrament of communion, where bread and wine (or juice) are used as symbols of the body and blood of Christ. However, the Seventh Day Adventists, members of the Church of Jesus Christ of the Latter-day Saints, and adherents of the Eastern Orthodox Church are unique in having a number of dietary practices intimately associated with their religious beliefs.

Seventh Day Adventists number almost 7 million worldwide. The Seventh Day Adventists Church had its early beginnings during the early part of the nineteenth century, when a worldwide interdenominational movement developed. Its followers were convinced that the second coming of Christ was near. In the United States, this movement was led by William Miller. The Seventh Day Adventists developed from a segment of his followers (Millerites) and was officially organized in 1863.

One of Miller's converts, Ellen Harmon, who later married James White, an Adventist preacher, had a very important influence on the church, including its views toward diet and health. She is said to have experienced over 2,000 prophetic visions and dreams, which she described in more than 100,000 hand-written manuscript pages. Many of her writings have been compiled into books, some of which relate to diet and health (White 1905; 1938). Seventh Day Adventists believe that the body is the temple of the Holy Spirit, as taught in the Scriptures (I Corinthians 3:16–17), and that "whether you eat or drink, or whatever you do, do all to the glory of God" (I Corinthians 10:31).

In 1863, Mrs. White wrote of a vision she experienced, which later was to have a profound effect on the dietary habits of Adventists. In the vision, she recognized that it was a sacred duty to attend to one's health and to "arouse others" to do so as well. Her vision convinced her that followers should come out against intemperance of every kind, in working, eating, drinking, and drugging, and to point people to God's great medicine, water. In her vision, she became aware of the importance of pure, soft water for diseases, for health, for cleanliness, and for luxury. Soon after, the first of many worldwide institutions dedicated to health was established by the church. Called the Western Health Reform Institute, it later became the world-reknowned Battle Creek Sanitarium in Battle Creek, Michigan.

The Seventh Day Adventists believe that good health is a treasure and that violating the laws of health will lead to sickness. One should maintain and preserve health through eating the right kinds of foods in moderation and by getting a sufficient amount of exercise and rest.

The church has a prohibition against eating the flesh (and fat) of unclean animals, as outlined in the Old Testament Scriptures. A vegetarian diet is recommended; however, it is not required for membership. About 40 to 50 percent of members are vegetarians. Although some adherents within this group consume no meat, milk, or eggs, most are lacto-ovo-vegetarians. The remaining 50 to 60 percent of Adventists eat meat, but usually much less than the general population (Bosley and Hardinge 1992:112). Stimulants such as tea and coffee are forbidden, as well as liquor and tobacco. Water is considered to be the best beverage, especially if it is soft. It should be drunk at room temperature, either before or after, but never during a meal. Spices are avoided. Eating between meals is discouraged in order to allow the digestive tract sufficient time to digest and absorb the food eaten at mealtimes. For the same reason, Mrs. White recommended that five to six hours should elapse between meals.

The Church of Jesus Christ of the Latter-day Saints (LDS) has a world-wide membership of over 8 million. It was founded in 1830 by Joseph Smith, the son of a New England farmer, and his associates. Its followers consider Smith to have been a modern prophet. They are called Mormons, because of their belief in the Book of Mormon, written and published by Smith in 1830.

Oscar Pike (1992:118) states that "Central to the dietary and health practices of members of the Church is a belief in continuing guidance from God through inspired leaders. In addition to the Bible and the Book of Mormon . . . church members accept as holy scripture instructions from God since the founding of the Church in 1830." These "latter-day" instructions are compiled in a book called the Doctrine and Covenants, which contains a simple health code (Section 89). This section concerns aspects of the diet and health of faithful members. It prohibits the use of tobacco products and the consumption of alcohol and "hot drinks," meaning coffee and tea. It further advises that meat should be used in moderation and emphasizes the use of fruit and grains.

According to Pike, a connection was made, some time ago, between the caffeine present in coffee and tea and their proscription. Thus, while not specifically forbidden by church doctrine, many church members avoid consuming all beverages containing caffeine. Because Mormons believe that the body serves as a "temple" for the spirit, there also is an emphasis on regular exercise and the avoidance of abusive substances.

The church encourages occasional fasting. Adherents are asked to fast once each month, usually the first Sunday, and to donate the money thus

saved as a "fast offering" for the poor. This monthly fast involves abstinence from food and drink for two consecutive meals.

The consumption of milk, frozen desserts, and water is higher among
Mormons than among non-LDS. Beverages which are caffeine- and alco-
hol-free are in demand. Utah, whose population is 70 percent Mormon,
has a per capita consumption of candy that is twice that of the rest of the
country. Also, considerable sugar is used for the making of home-made
sweets and in baking and canning. Mormons tend to eat at home.

The eating habits of Mormons are similar to those of the Adventists in
a number of ways. Both groups teach abstinence from tea, coffee, alcohol,
and tobacco. Both emphasize the consumption of plant products and plenty
of water. Both LDS and Adventists view the human body as a temple not
to be defiled by poor diets and unnecessary drugs. Regular exercise is encouraged. The lifestyle of these two groups is believed to be an essential
factor in their lower mortality rates and greater longevity, as well as decreased incidence of cancer, heart disease, alcoholism, cirrhosis, and other
diseases.

The Eastern Orthodox Church. This group has about 170 million members worldwide. Orthodox Christian churches were established in the Holy
Lands before Christianity spread to Rome. But by A.D. 300, the two principal centers of Christianity were Rome and Constantinople, and they had
already begun to compete with one another for absolute power and authority over all Christians. In A.D. 1054, this power struggle culminated in
a division of the followers of Christianity into the Church of Rome and
the Eastern Orthodox Church, headquartered at Constantinople (now Is-
tanbul).

The Greek Orthodox religion includes many diet-related practices, including numerous fast days and feast days (see Kittler and Sucher 1989:
31–33). On fast days, all meat and animal products are forbidden,
including milk, butter, and cheese. Fish also is taboo, with the exception
of shellfish (such as clams, shrimp, and oysters). Every fast day is supposed
to be a day of sexual abstinence. Meals of dried bean and lentil soup are
commonly consumed on fast days in Greece.

Easter is the most important holiday event in the Eastern Orthodox
Church. It occurs on the first Sunday after the full moon which occurs on
or immediately after March 21, but it may not precede the Jewish Passover.
The 40-day Lent period is preceded by a three-week pre-Lenten period of
preparation and repentance. The third Sunday before Lent (Meat Fare Sunday), all the meat in the house is consumed. On the Sunday before Lent
(Cheese Fare Sunday), all cheese, eggs, and butter in the house are consumed. On the next day, "Clean Monday," the family is ready to begin
the true Great Lent and abstain from all animal foods until Easter Sunday.
Fish is allowed only on Palm Sunday and the Annunciation Day of the
Virgin Mary. Lentil soup is always eaten on Good Friday to symbolize the

tears of the Virgin Mary. The lentil soup often is served with vinegar, in remembrance of Christ's having been given vinegar on the cross instead of the water he requested.

The Orthodox Easter fast traditionally is broken after the midnight Resurrection Service on Easter Sunday with mageritsa, a soup made with the internal organs of the lamb such as the tripe, liver, pancreas, lungs, and heart. Lamb is the traditional food on Easter. Another traditional Greek custom is the baking of thick, round, leaven loaves of Easter bread decorated with colored, hard-boiled eggs. The eggs are always dyed bright red, symbolic of the blood of Christ which redeemed the world. The breaking open of these eggs on Easter morning symbolizes the opening of the tomb of Christ and is an outward sign of belief in the resurrection of Christ. One person cracks his egg against the egg of another, saying *"Christos Anesti"* (Christ is risen); the other person replies *"Alithos Anestia"* (Indeed, he is risen) (Lowenberg et al. 1979:172–73).

Judaism

This religion has about 18 million followers worldwide. It is one of the world's oldest major religions. The ancestors of the Hebrews were seminomads roving the lands of Egypt, Syria, and Mesopotamia about 2000 B.C. It was the first religion to teach the belief in one God. Unlike the other major religions, Judaism is the religion of only one people—the Jews. Both Christianity and Islam developed from Judaism. These religions accept the Jewish belief in one God and the moral teachings of the Hebrew Bible (which in modified form Christians call the Old Testament). Judaism teaches that all people are created in the image of God and deserve to be treated with dignity and respect. Thus, moral and ethical teaching play a more important role in Judaism than do teachings about God.

Dietary laws. Kashrut, the Jewish laws governing food and its preparation are based on the Torah (the first five books of the Hebrew Bible) and the Laws of Kashrut, contained in the Talmud, a later sacred writing. Although these dietary laws are still practiced by many orthodox Jews as part of their religious beliefs, not all Jewish people today observe these traditional dietary habits.

According to Carol Bryant et al. (1985:216–17), Jewish dietary laws can be divided into three components. First, all animal and vegetable components of food must be derived from approved species, as outlined in the Torah (particularly Leviticus, chapter 2, and Deuteronomy, chapter 14) and the Laws of Kashrut. Approved animal species include four-footed animals that both ruminate (chew cud) and have cloven hooves, birds that do not eat carrion, and fish with scales. All other animals, as well as their milk and eggs, are forbidden. These include swine (which have cloven hooves but do not chew cud), the rabbit and camel (which chew cud but do not have cloven hooves), as well as carnivores, rodents, shellfish, birds of prey, eaters of carrion, and reptiles. Most plant species are approved.

A second element of Jewish dietary law requires that approved species must be prepared correctly. Warm-blooded animals must be ritually slaughtered. A rabbi must be present at all such slaughterings, which are carried out by a trained person called a *shokhet*. The animal must be killed in a manner that ensures a minimum of pain. The shokhet's blade must be so sharp that one swift, deep, almost painless slash at the throat of the animal renders it almost immediately unconscious and allows the blood to drain from its body as completely as possible. Blood is considered a sacred substance, and its consumption is strictly forbidden (Leviticus 17:11). Therefore, any remaining blood must be removed from the slaughtered animal by ritual soaking. The internal fat of an animal also is taboo. Thus, only those soaps and scouring powders that do not contain animal fats may be used for washing dishes. Detergents are permitted.

The meat from animals so slaughtered is carefully inspected and then stamped with the seal of the shokhet to indicate its ritual purity. Such approved foods are designated as *"kosher."*

The third general dietary ruling is that milk and all dairy products must not be mixed with meat products. The admonition against mixing meat and dairy foods seems to be based on three statements in Exodus and in Deuteronomy that warn adherents not to "seethe the kid in the milk of its mother." Although the basis of this proscription is unclear, it may have stemmed from the increased possibility of meat spoilage when mixed with milk, since the latter is such an excellent medium for bacterial growth, especially at warm Middle Eastern temperatures.

Thus, *kosher* dietary laws define which plant and animal species can be eaten, how they should be prepared, and what food categories can be consumed together. In addition to the Jewish Sabbath, there are numerous other Jewish religious holidays (Figures 8.1 and 8.2). Jews also observe several fast days, including Yom Kippur, a complete fast day (no food or water) (Kittler and Sucher 1989:24–29). (For more information regarding Jewish dietary practices, see also Lowenberg et al. 1979; Regenstein and Regenstein 1979.)

Jewish congregations in the United States generally are classified as Orthodox, Conservative, or Reform. Although all the groups agree on most matters of basic theology, they differ in their interpretation of the ancient rituals and the need to practice them. Orthodox Jews perceive that the ancient dietary practices and rituals are directives from God, which demand strict adherence. Reform Jews conform to them the least. Conservative Jews represent a middle ground between Orthodox and Reform beliefs.

Although practicing the Laws of Kashrut made it more difficult for Jews to relate to Gentiles, and tended to set them apart, it also provided Jews with a strong sense of identity and solidarity. Although Reform Jews feel

Figure 8.2
First Night of Passover

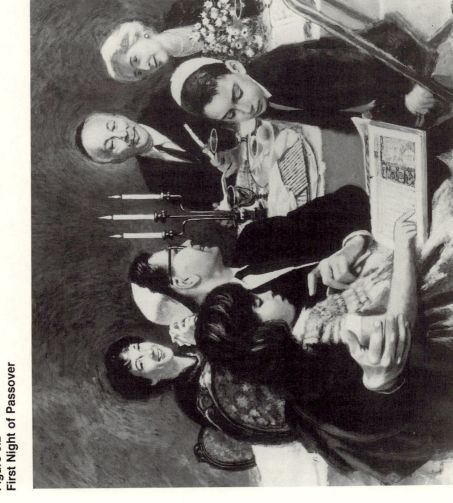

Orthodox Jewish family observing the first night of Passover. Courtesy of the B. Manischewitz Company, Jersey City, N.J.

that customs that reflect religious principles should change with the times, many of them feel a sense of loss from the discontinuation of certain traditional rituals. But Reform Jews have not yet introduced any new customs to take their place (see Future Role of Food in Religion, below).

Islam

The youngest and second largest of the major world religions, Islam now is both a religion and way of life for over 971 million people. It was founded in Saudi Arabia in A.D. 622 by the prophet Mohammed. Mohammed had come in contact with both Jews and Christians during his early years. He was impressed with their belief in one god, in contrast with the many gods of his fellow Arabians.

Mohammed taught that there was only one God, Allah, and that all must submit completely to his will. The word *Islam* means submission, and the word *Muslim* means "one who submits." Muslims perceive the God of Judaism, of Christianity, and of Islam to be basically the same, because all three religions trace their origins back to the early Hebrews through Abraham (Genesis:16). However, Muslims believe that the word of Allah was incompletely expressed in the Old and New testaments, and was only fulfilled in the Koran, the most sacred writing of Islam (Kittler and Sucher 1989:37).

The religious practices of the followers of Islam are known as the Five Pillars of Islam. The first four pillars are faith, prayer, alms, and fasting. The last pillar of Islam is the pilgrimage, or *haji*, to Mecca, the goal of every devout Muslim.

Dietary practices. There is much emphasis on fasting for God's sake, including the mandatory fast of Ramadan. There also are several feast days (Kittler and Sucher 1989:40–41).

In view of Mohammed's early contact with both Judaism and Christianity, it is understandable that Islam reflects traditional Judeo-Christian principles and shares many of the Jewish dietary restrictions. The Koran, like the Jewish Torah and Talmud, instructs followers as to which foods are considered to be clean and proper, and how they should be eaten. Animals that die of disease, strangulation, or beating are forbidden (law of carrion). Blood is forbidden, as well as swine (pork). Four passages in the Koran forbid the eating of pork. No animal food except fish and locusts is considered lawful unless it has been slaughtered according to the approved ritual, which is similar to that of the Jewish shokhet. The person killing the animal must repeat at the instant of slaughter, "In the name of God, God is great." Muslims must also abstain from drinking wine or other intoxicating beverages (Lowenberg et al., 1979:184). Smoking and the use of tea and coffee are discouraged. Nevertheless, many Muslims indulge in these activities.

Hinduism

Thought to be the oldest living religion, Hinduism originated in India about 4,000 years ago. Its followers currently number approximately 733 million worldwide. The vast majority of Hindus live in the Indian subcontinent.

Arun Kilara and K. K. Iya (1992:94) have observed that, though it has a singular name, the manifestations of the Hindu religion are many. C.C. Joseph (1974) has pointed out that Hinduism is a synthesis of diverse and competing faiths. The latter include monistic, monotheistic, polytheistic, pantheistic, animistic, totemistic, agnostic, and even atheistic beliefs. Therefore, Hinduism embodies a tolerant and forebearing philosophy that is hard to define. Nevertheless, certain generalizations can be made.

To the non-Hindu, it may appear that Hindus worship numerous deities. However, there is only one supreme being, known as Brahman, and the various gods worshipped by Hindus simply are manifestations of him.

The supreme authority for Hinduism is contained in the four eternal books called Vedas: Rig, Yajur, Sama, and Atharva. The caste system, or *varanas*, is described in the Vedas, and, therefore, is institutionalized in religion. It is very intimately involved in the Hindu way of life and religion.

Dietary practices. Definite rules and regulations exist for members of each caste. Dietary restrictions and attitudes vary among the castes and serve as a means of distinguishing among them. Kilara and Iya (1992:94) have noted that distinctions among castes always have been easy to demonstrate through rules of eating. Violations of these rules are taken seriously, since they pose a threat to social order and the individual's sense of identity.

In 1949, through the efforts of Mohandas Gandhi, the Indian government expressed opposition to the social barriers of caste. However, since social changes of this nature are accepted slowly, the caste system still is a powerful influence, particularly in the villages.

The Hindu believes that nothing that once existed is ever completely destroyed; it merely undergoes a change in its form. The orthodox Hindu believes that, since all living things contain part of the divine spirit of Brahman, all life is sacred. Therefore, taking the life of a living creature is akin to harming Brahman. The Hindu's belief in reincarnation further reinforces the Hindu law against killing any living thing, since one could never be certain that it did not contain the soul of an ancestor reborn as the animal.

The Code of Manu, a sacred Hindu writing, contains many laws governing the diet of the Hindu. Most members of the Brahmin caste are strict vegetarians who follow the nonviolent attitude and strict rules of the Code of Manu. The members of the other castes may eat meat other than beef, but the higher the caste, the greater the prejudice against this practice. Beef is especially taboo, since the cow is perceived as a particularly sacred animal. Many anthropologists believe that the cow's special status derives from its having been of greater value to the family, alive, as a beast of burden and ongoing source of milk and cheese for food, and dung for fuel, than slaughtered and consumed as a source of meat. In addition to meat, especially beef, the Code of Manu forbids to the higher castes the eating of domestic fowls, onions, garlic, turnips, mushrooms, and salted pork. Blood is expressly forbidden. Both fasting and feasting are important components of Hindu dietary practices (see Kittler and Sucher 1989:46–47).

Buddhism

This religion is an outgrowth of Hinduism and currently has a membership of 315 million worldwide. In 250 B.C., Buddhism was made India's state religion. Today, less than 1 percent of India's population is Buddhist. Most Buddhists now live in Sri Lanka, the mainland nations of Southeast Asia, and Japan. Originating during the sixth century B.C., it was founded by Siddhartha Gautama, who was to become Buddha—the Enlightened One.

Gautama was raised as a Hindu, the son of a wealthy Himalayan chieftain. At the age of 29, deeply concerned with the misery and suffering of humanity, he gave up his worldly goods and became a beggar. He wandered throughout northeast India, meditating and seeking the answer to the dilemma of human suffering. After six years, he experienced enlightenment. He became convinced that, finally, he had discovered the reason for human misery and how people could escape it. For the rest of his life, he traveled throughout India, teaching the Eight-fold Path. By following the Eight-fold Path, one is cured of selfish desires, the cause of suffering. It involves practicing right belief, right thought, right speech, right action, right means of livelihood, right exertion, right remembrance, and right meditation.

Dietary practices. Certain aspects of the Eight-fold Path relate to food habits, particularly the right action and the right livelihood. The right action is interpreted to include abstention from taking a life. Therefore, the killing and eating of living creatures is forbidden. The right action also includes the eating of what are considered the "right foods," which, essentially, means vegetarian foods. Growing rice and other crops is regarded as the "right livelihood" because it does not entail the taking of a life. Production of livestock for meat consumption would be forbidden.

Buddhist food practices vary considerably with the sect and country of residence. Because of the proscription against the taking of life, many followers are lacto-ovo-vegetarians. However, others abstain only from beef. Some Buddhists eat fish. Some monks may fast twice a month, on the days of the new and full moon. Buddhist festivals vary by regions. However, most Buddhists celebrate *pravarana*, the end of the rainy season (Kittler and Sucher 1989:49–50).

ORIGINS OF DIETARY PRACTICES

It can be seen from the foregoing discussion of dietary practices, that all of the five major religions prohibit some food, either completely or at certain times. In every case, these foods are of animal origin. Traditionally, for certain groups within Hindu society and for Buddhists, no meat of any kind should be eaten. For all Hindu castes, beef is especially tabooed. The eating of pork or blood is proscribed for both Orthodox Jews and Muslims. Hindus also are forbidden to consume blood, as well as eggs. Catholics are forbidden to eat fish on the Fridays of Lent; if members of the Eastern Orthodox Church abstain faithfully from meat, fish, and dairy products on all of the designated fast days, these foods are not eaten on about 186 days out of the year. Why this proscription of animal foods?

Unquestionably, an important factor must be the disapproval of meat eating by several religions because it involves the taking of life. Many scholars believe that existing dietary habits, familiar to the people, often came to be perceived as the "right habits" and so may have become prescribed as such by religious leaders. For example, if animal meat were scarce, plant foods would become the customary food, which later came to be perceived as the "acceptable" food. Also, in times of meat scarcity, forbidding meat by church leaders may have served the pragmatic purpose of conserving a scarce food commodity. Conversely, foods which were unfamiliar, or consumed by the enemy, might come to be regarded with distaste or disapproval.

The widespread proscription of the pig frequently has raised questions. Frederick Simoons (1961) has suggested that the original prejudice against the pig developed among the pastoral people living in the arid regions of Asia. The pig was not commonly eaten by members of their group but was raised and consumed by the sedentary agriculturists in the area. There was always competition between the two groups for existing land, and the resultant ill feeling may have led to contempt for the rival group's food, as well. Once the prejudice was established, it may then have become incorporated into the sacred writings. It is interesting that the pig is forbidden, not only for Jews and Muslims, but for Hindus and Buddhists as well.

FUTURE ROLE OF FOOD IN RELIGION

Since primitive times, human beings have used food as a means of relating to a supreme being. Since food is so essential to physical existence, it is not surprising that it became imbued with religious significance. Along with their religious role, dietary habits (perhaps coincidentally) have served as a means of separating one religious group from another. This circumstance has had particular significance for minority groups at risk for becoming absorbed into a larger culture (e.g., the Jews, as they led their nomadic existence). In such situations, the retention of special dietary habits served to maintain the identity of the smaller group and to provide a common bond among its members, in turn strengthening their religious beliefs.

However, over the years, especially in modern times, religious dietary habits often have been relaxed or discontinued. As a consequence, many adherents have expressed a feeling of loss.

What of the future? If the role of food in religion continues to decrease, will people need to obtain the spiritual gratification they once received from the observance of certain religious dietary practices from another source? If so, will it involve new food habits or rituals? During the past 15 to 20 years, many Americans, especially young people, have explored alternative food practices, including some which are associated with Eastern religions. Some observers perceive these dietary innovations (at times ritualistic) as attempts to find meaning and security and to fill the existing void with respect to the symbolic use of food. Others have speculated that the current zealous interest in diet and fitness (with its ritualistic behaviors) also may, in part, represent a search for security and increased meaning in life.

Campbell (1988) believed that the Judeo-Christian mythologies, originating in the first millennium, now are outdated. He felt that new ones are needed, but that change, especially during the twentieth century, has occurred so fast that they have not yet had a chance to develop and mature. Myths are most likely to develop in a slow-moving, postfigurative society.

FOR FURTHER READING

Bosley, G.C., and M.G. Hardinge. 1992. Seventh-day Adventists: dietary standards and concerns. *Food Technology* 46(10):112–13.

Campbell, J. 1988. *The power of myth*. New York: Doubleday.

Chaudry, M.M. 1992. Islamic food laws: philosophic basis and practical implications. *Food Technology* 46(10):92–93, 104.

Kilara, A., and K.K. Iya. 1991. Food and dietary habits of the Hindu. *Food Technology* 46(10):94–104.

Kittler, P., and K. Sucher. 1989. *Food and culture in America*. New York: Van Nostrand Reinhold.

La Farge, O. 1956. *A pictorial history of the American Indian*. New York: Crown Publishers.

Lowenberg, M.D., E.N. Todhunter, E.D. Wilson, J.R. Savage, and J.L. Lubawski. 1979. *Food and people* (3rd ed.). New York: John Wiley and Sons.

Nash, M. 1963. Burmese Buddhism in everyday life. *American Anthropologist* 65: 285.

Pike, O.A. 1992. The Church of Jesus Christ of Latter Day Saints: dietary practices and health. *Food Technology* 46(10):118–21.

Rice, E. 1973. *The five great religions*. New York: Four Winds Press.

Figure 9.1
Preparing Belgian Trippe for Folk Fest Visitors

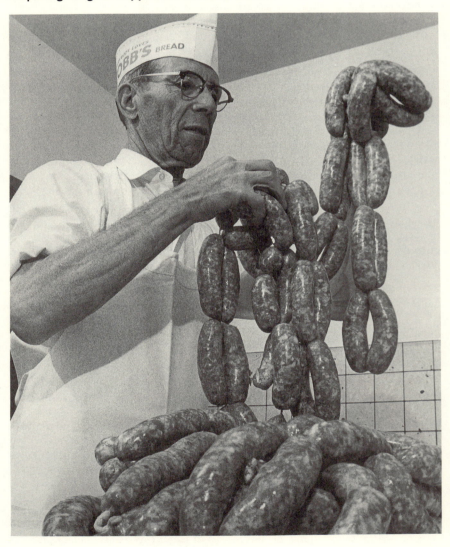

The Neville Public Museum of Brown County

9

American Food: A Characterization

American food consists of mainstream cuisine (regular home cooking), regional dishes (including "regional phenomena"), and "pop" food (including fast food). Before exploring the characteristics of these types of American cuisine, let us examine the cultural (and other) influences which have made it what it is today.

EARLY INFLUENCES

The Native Americans

The history of American food begins with the native American Indians, who had occupied the Western Hemisphere thousands of years before the arrival of the white man. In early encounters with them, early European explorers found that the Indian natives were farmers as well as hunter-gatherers. They were adept both at raising crops and procuring game.

The early settlers on the Eastern Seaboard learned a great deal from the Indian regarding obtaining and preparing the unfamiliar foods upon which they now had to rely heavily for sustenance. As the settlers moved to the south and west, the Indians there also made valuable contributions to their pioneer cuisines. In short, the Indian has exerted a far greater influence on the foodways of what became the United States than is generally recognized.

The Indians could claim only one staple: corn. But they made excellent use of this staple in a variety of dishes, which colonists adapted and modified. They included corn pone, hoe cake, hominy (including grits), corn sticks, johnnycake, "buckskin bread," spoon bread, and hush puppies. Corn also was used to make soups and stews. The colonists learned that beans, another common crop of the Indians, could be combined with corn to make succotash and samp. Squash was another important vegetable, which the Europeans recognized as similar to those available in their homeland. Squash and pumpkin were especially popular with the northeastern Indians, baked and served with some sort of animal fat, maple syrup, or honey. Pumpkin, when made into a soup, was boiled with meat until it became more like a stew, according to a seventeenth-century Oneida recipe (Root and de Rochemont 1976:40).

Other foods introduced by the Indians, and refined by early settlers, were wild rice, baked beans, Indian pudding, maple sugar, pinto beans, and chili peppers. "Hog 'n' hominy," that special combination of salt pork and corn, is credited with keeping the pioneers alive in every phase of the westward migration (Jones 1990:8). Although the Indians made great use of vegetables, the greater share of the Indian diet was provided by game. The Indian taught the settlers how (and where) to hunt and fish locally and also the rudiments of food preservation. Drying was especially popular, not only for beans and corn, two of their most important foods, but also for meat. From the Indians the pioneers learned to make jerky and pemmican (packets of ground, dried meat, fat, berries, and occasionally dried bone marrow). These foods were important to the pioneers as they opened up the Far West.

The main beverage of the Indian was water, augmented by significant amounts of tea, made from sassafras, wild mint, or sumac berries. The settlers did not introduce the Indian to alcohol. Like peoples the world over, they already were familiar with fermentation processes which occurred naturally in sugar-containing foods, especially fruit juices (see chapter 2). There are accounts of wine that was made from wild grapes; wine is commonly included in the long list of foods thought to have been served at the first Thanksgiving feast at Plymouth, in 1621. However, the Indians of the Northeast had not yet learned to distill fermented alcoholic beverages to make hard liquor.

Along with their contributions to staples, the Indians added special "accents" in their cooking, which were adopted also by the settlers. One of their techniques was the use of filé, particularly by the Choctaw, a powder made of dried, pounded sassafras leaves. This gray-green powder was used to thicken soups and stews, and later, in the preparation of gumbo, which Africans had introduced in the South. Other substances, used by the Seminole Indians, were comfortroot (for making flour), and the sometimes mouth-puckering persimmon, both of which required special handling. The

Indians generally made wide use of fruits in many of their dishes, including some borrowed from the Europeans. Cranberry sauce originated with the Indians; they may also have introduced the first cobbler, with their practice of adding blackberries or strawberries to cornmeal dough (Root and de Rochemont 1976:29, 38).

Indians in the Southeast are credited with developing Brunswick stew. There were no fixed ingredients but included anything and everything (except fish): usually corn and beans (like succotash) and game, especially squirrel, rabbit, and turkey. Today, it is made from chicken and vegetables.

The Indians contributed to both Creole and to Cajun cooking. Indian foods, especially corn dishes, have been very important to the development of all of the regions of the United States.

The Spaniards

The Spanish became the first colonizers in America when Columbus brought 1,500 settlers to the island of Hispaniola in the West Indies on his second voyage in 1493. He also brought along cuttings of sugar cane to the Western Hemisphere on this voyage, as well as orange seeds. This island became a base for further Spanish expansion into other parts of the Western Hemisphere.

During the 1500s, the Spanish conquered the Inca of Peru, the Maya of Central America and the Aztecs of Mexico. By 1600, Spain and Portugal (who now controlled Brazil) ruled most of the hemisphere from Mexico southward. During the 1500s, the Spaniards also moved into what is now the southeastern and western United States. They took control of Florida, the Gulf Rim, and the land west of the Mississippi River. The Spanish began to demonstrate an undeniable presence on the mainland of North America with the establishment of the first permanent European settlement at St. Augustine, Florida, in 1565. Missions and other settlements in the South and West followed. Except for a 40-year period of French rule, the Spanish were in command of this area until the Louisiana Territory was taken over by the United States in 1803.

Along with their physical presence, the Spaniards exerted an early culinary influence on American cooking. These colonizers had discovered chocolate from the Aztecs and introduced it to North America and Europe. Hernando de Soto is known to have planted oranges in Florida by 1539. They are thought to have been the bitter orange, which grows wild in Florida today. The sweet orange came later and today is almost synonymous with the state (Root and de Rochemont 1976:47).

The Spanish are credited with being the first to bring several important animals over to North America, first to the West Indies and then to the mainland (Florida). Some of them arrived in San Domingo in 1493 on Columbus's second voyage, one of the most important of which has to be the chicken. The first domestic hogs of North America are thought to be thirteen pigs introduced in Florida in 1542 by Hernando de Soto, to supply a base near Tampa. Cattle were brought ashore in Florida at least by 1550. Texas got its cattle a little later—animals which had escaped from the conquistadors. These contributions were not uniquely Spanish, since the British also brought over chickens, cattle, and hogs to the English colonies to the north (Root and de Rochemont 1976:46).

The Spanish had begun to produce sugar in the Caribbean by 1516 (Mintz 1991:117). Sugar cane was brought to Louisiana by Jesuit missionaries in 1751, and the first sugar mill on the North American mainland began operating in New Orleans in 1791 (Wyse 1989:961).

The Spanish welcomed the new condiments which they found in the Caribbean. Columbus and his men encountered over 200 kinds of peppers there, ranging from the bell pepper to the hot chilies (Jones 1990:64–68). There was a flow of foods and condiments from South and Central America via the West Indies toward Florida. In addition, there also was transferral of Latin American foods and condiments up the western side of the Gulf Coast, from Mexico and further south, to the Spanish settlements along the western Gulf fringe. The Spaniards soon incorporated some of these foods and spices as "accent pieces" into their cuisine, which later has become part of American cooking. Although not completely unique to them, they have become part of the characteristic "flavor" of Spanish cooking. These include the chilies, olives, capers, *comino* (cumin), oregano, and dried safflower blossoms (used as a substitute for the expensive saffron of the Old World). Others had been first encountered in the New World, borrowed from the Southwest Indian and added to their own dishes: pumpkin seeds, *yerba buena* (which grew wild on the hills above San Francisco Bay), and piñon nuts (Jones 1990:59–80). The unique chili flavor was introduced into the Spanish style of cooking that prevailed in the Southwest before the region was taken over by the United States.

The exotic fruits growing in Florida were welcomed by the Spanish. Later, the avocado, pineapple, and coconuts arrived.

In the Southwest, the European influence on food was of Spanish origin, along with Aztec and other Indian overtones. In the Southeast and in Florida, particularly, the Continental Spanish influence had been modified by the produce of tropical islands. Spanish cooking developed into what is known as Creole cuisine along the rim of the Gulf of Mexico (Jones 1990: 59–60).

Like other Europeans, Spaniards planted the seeds and encouraged the appetite for beans, especially the red ones that are often kidney shaped, known in Spanish as *frijoles colorados* or *habichuelas*. Red beans and rice is a basic dish as typical of southern Louisiana as is Hoppin' John (black-eyed peas and rice) of the Carolinas. While beans are not completely unique to the Spanish, they constitute an intrinsic component of Spanish-influenced

American food. In addition to the beans used by the Indians, the conquistadors also brought black beans into Florida from the Caribbean islands and imported garbanzos (chick peas) from the Old World (Jones 1990:60–62). Black beans and rice are sometimes used for a party dish in Ybor City, the cigar-making suburb of Tampa.

Rum was brought to the mainland to Florida from Puerto Rico by Ponce de Leon, a hundred years before the first European settlement. In addition to its use as a beverage, rum was used by the Spaniards to accent the oregano and garlic flavors of black beans.

It was through the Spanish that the avocado (native to Central and South America) was introduced to Florida and California. It had been grown for years in the Spanish missions of California. By 1924, Anglo farmers were growing it seriously enough to organize the Avocado Growers Exchange. Now both California and Florida export the fruits to markets around the world (Jones 1990:70–71).

A Spanish dish with an Aztec component, very popular in California, is turkey *mole*. It is a complex mixture of ground turkey and many seasonings, to which bitter chocolate also is added. Another dish with both Indian and Spanish origins is *menudo* (from the Spanish, meaning entrails). It is sometimes described as a New World–Old World dish, since it is made with New World hominy (Indian) and Old World tripe (Spanish). For years, it has been a traditional Christmas breakfast dish among Spanish Americans.

Some of the most important contributions of the Spaniards to American cooking include the use of peppers, garlic, olives, oranges, pomegranates, and wine (which developed from efforts of the grape-growing Spanish priests, in California), chorizo, and jambalaya. Although the Spanish did not invent the barbecue, they perhaps deserve credit for the name. The Spanish word *barbacoa* was applied by early Spanish explorers to the outdoor grilling of meat by the Indians of Haiti. The colonizers of the Southwest refined this practice and Anglicized the Spanish term for it to "barbecue." Today it is a popular method of preparing meat, not only in the Southwest, but throughout the country.

The Spanish have influenced the evolution of American cooking more than is generally recognized. Evan Jones believes that there probably are more Spanish flavors in American food than other European influences (78).

The African Slaves

Although some of today's food writers ignore the African influence on American foodways, African cooking has had a tremendous impact on American eating habits. The year 1619 marked the introduction of Africans to the American colonies, when the first African laborers were delivered to

Virginia (Jernegan 1959:87). Thus began an influx of Africans to the colonies that went on for almost 250 years. The coming of slaves enriched the repertoire of available foods in the colonies because the Africans carried seeds with them to the New World. The black-eyed pea, so popular in the South today, was introduced in this fashion in 1674; okra and watermelon were others.

Gumbo or okra has to be one of the more well-known African influences on American cuisine, especially that of the Gulf rim, including Louisiana. Gumbo comes from the African work *kinggombo* or *kingumbo*—meaning okra. After its introduction, the use of okra spread throughout the South westward along the Gulf Coast to Louisiana. The African slaves, like the Indians, have contributed to both Creole and Cajun cooking.

The Middle Passage. Historian O. P. Chitwood has described this facet of the English slave trade:

But, in 1697, the right to share in this [the English slave trade] was allowed all British subjects, and in the 18th Century, a good many American ships, mostly from New England were engaged in the slave trade. The New England merchants linked up the slave trade with the manufacture and sale of rum in such a way as to make the combined business quite profitable. Rum was shipped from New England to the west Coast of Africa, and bartered for Negroes. These were taken to the West Indies and exchanged for molasses and other commodities. From the molasses brought back to the home ports was manufactured the rum that was used as cargo on the first part of the three-sided voyage, which was known as the "three-cornered" or "triangular" trade. The trip from Africa to the West
Indies was called the "Middle Passage," as it was . . . the second or middle lap of the triangular voyage. (Chitwood 1961:345)

Foods of the Middle Passage. "Slave traders, interested in ensuring that as much of their lucrative cargo survived the middle passage as possible, may have been inadvertently responsible for the transportation of yams, as well as numerous other indigenous African crops to the Americas. By at least the early 1700s, slavers had learned that, although some English foods were acceptable, slaves fared better when fed their customary food" (Hall 1991:163). Yams, rice, corn, melegueta pepper and palm oil, and peanuts (depending on their area of origin) were made available during the passage. Robert Hall has described in detail the links between the Atlantic slave trade and the dispersal of yams, millet and sorghum, rice, bananas, citrus fruits, corn, cassava, and melegueta pepper to North America (162–67).

Although scholars today recognize the importance of the introduction of African plants to North America by the Africans, the European slave traders of the time valued them from another standpoint. They knew that the slaves were familiar with the cultivation of grains and realized the potential value of obtaining workers already equipped with agrarian skills, so essential on the American plantations (Hall 1991:166).

It was fortunate that most plantation owners allowed the slaves to have small plots on which to raise gardens. In this way, their food supply was increased, and their nutrition frequently surpassed that of the planters themselves (Olmsted 1860). In addition, with the seeds they carried with them, they were able to propagate and perpetuate their Old World cooking styles.

The house servants, especially, were able to augment their diets by utilizing parts of vegetables and meats discarded during the preparation of foods in the masters' kitchens. The slaves became adept at utilizing discarded portions of vegetables (leaves or stems, as the case might be) and such leftover animal parts as pig knuckles, hocks, pig's feet, snout, jowl, haws, and intestines. In cooking this meat, they used generous portions of the spices with which they were already familiar. The collective cuisine that evolved from these practices has been revived during the past 20 years, as part of a general ethnic revival in the United States, some of it known as soul food.

The Africans had a particularly strong influence on Southern cooking, because of the greater population of slaves in the South. It is obvious that slave cooks introduced some of their foods and favorite dishes to the white planters, and that, gradually, they found their way into accepted Southern cuisine.

Like religion, oral traditions, music, dance, and material culture, cuisine and culinary practices not only survived Africans' capture, the middle passage, and hard servitude but also enriched the cultures of the Americas. Fried chicken, among other southern dishes, reflects this African influence; even the seasoning of southern dishes, often far heavier than in northern recipes, constitutes another African influence. When Americans of any hue sit down to a meal of gumbo, spicy chicken garnished with peanuts (goobers), black-eyed peas or pigeon peas and rice, cola, and dessert of banana pudding or yam pie sweetened with sorghum molasses, we are savoring a taste of Africa. The vitality of these culinary traditions in the Americas is a testament to the richness of African cultures and to those Africans who shared that richness with their [surrounding] societies. (Hall 1991:161)

To most readers, this hypothetical dinner described by Hall will appear to be stereotypically American. Its familiarity demonstrates the extent to which African food habits have been assimilated into American cuisine. "To the extent that it reflects mutual acculturation, the African and American culinary exchange is representative of the cultural amalgamation that typifies the Columbian exchange" (169).

LATER INFLUENCES

The French

In 1541, Hernando de Soto led a group of explorers into the lower Mississippi River area in an unsuccessful quest for gold. But the Spaniards made no further explorations of this area after De Soto died in 1542.

In 1682, the French explorer René Robert Cavelier, Sieur de la Salle traveled down the Mississippi River. Upon reaching its mouth, he claimed the entire river valley for France, naming the region Louisiana in honor of the reigning French king, Louis XIV. Louisiana became a French royal colony in 1699, and French settlements followed. In 1718, Jean Baptiste le Moyne, Sieur de Bienville, the governor of Louisiana, founded New Orleans, on the east side of the Mississippi's mouth. In 1762, France ceded Louisiana to Spain, who ruled the area until 1800.

Also, when the English gained control of Canada, many French Canadians moved to the United States or were deported from Canada. Most of them settled in northern New England, especially Maine, where their descendants are known as Franco-Americans (Kittler and Sucher, 1989). About 4,000 French Canadians from Acadia (now Nova Scotia) fled to central and southern Louisiana between the 1760s and 1790. Their descendants now are called Cajuns.

The influence of these French settlers on American cuisine will be discussed later in this chapter.

Other Immigrants

Most of the colonists in the northeastern United States were English, with lesser numbers of Dutch, German, Scotch-Irish, Scottish and Swedes. During the early years of the Republic, land-hungry immigrants began pouring into America. With the first wave of immigration during the 1830s, 1840s, and 1850s, a substantial number of immigrants arrived, mainly from Germany, Great Britain, and Ireland. The second wave of immigrants, who arrived between 1860 and 1890, came mainly from German, Great Britain, Ireland, and the Scandinavian countries. The third wave, between 1890 and 1930, brought 22 million immigrants, mostly from Greece, Austria-Hungary, Italy, Poland, Portugal, Russia, and Spain (see Table 5.1). The greatest numbers were from Austria-Hungary, Italy, and Russia. Whereas these earlier immigrants came from Europe, a majority of immigrants coming to the United States within the past half-century have come from Southeast Asia, Latin America, and the Caribbean. All of these groups have contributed ethnic dishes to American cuisine to varying degrees.

MAINSTREAM CUISINE

The principal cuisines which have been integrated into American mainstream cooking are the British (they were the first true colonizers), the Dutch, and the German. Historically, Americans have been very conservative about allowing foods of other ethnic origins into the mainstream cuisine.

British Cooking

English cuisine has been described as possessing a forthrightness and simplicity with respect to their preparation of raw ingredients, an attribute not shared by the French. The kitchens with which the early British colonists were familiar had been rudimentary, open-hearthed, and equipped with only a spit or two for cooking meats. Therefore, they adapted relatively easily to the sparse equipment with which they worked in their New World homes. As soon as possible, colonists built log cabins with fireplaces; however, much early cooking was done outdoors, barbecue fashion, a universal method already familiar from Britain and also practiced by their new Indian neighbors (Figure 4.4). Initially, their modest utensils were ones brought with them by ship from England. Typically, they might consist of a few skillets, a frying pan, a small stewing pan, and a can for boiling pudding. Later, this food often was prepared in a cast-iron pot with a heavy, deep-edged iron cover, which sat on three short legs among the glowing (hot) fireplace coals (Jones 1990).

These early New England cooks developed good, plain dishes from the local foods available, prepared with such simple ingredients as butter and flour, and seasoned with a few spices or sweet herbs (Jones 1990:5). Most Englishmen felt the need for at least a modest number of spices. Those who could afford it bought pepper, cloves, mace, cinnamon, and ginger. Even the Pilgrims preferred such conventional seasonings, when they were available.

Contemporary observers have sometimes criticized Anglo cooking as unimaginative. True or not, the colonists were eating much as affluent Britons in their homeland were eating at that time. Like their British counterparts, New Englanders used vegetables primarily as sauces to accompany meats, rather than as substantial menu items. Green and leafy vegetables tended to be scorned (Levenstein 1988:4). By contrast, the Indians were enthusiastic vegetable eaters, and their example (as well as necessity) appears to have soon stimulated greater consumption of plant foods among the English.

At least by 1824, judging from Mary Randolph's cookbook, *The Virginia Housewife,* there had been some breaking away from the English past by successive generations of Anglos. Her cookbook was the first to devote an entire section to vegetables and to feature some not commonly served in England, such as sweet potatoes, pumpkin, squashes, and tomatoes. She also described various methods for preparing fresh, young turnip greens, by then considered a traditional southern dish (Jones 1990).

Dutch Cooking

Waverly Root and Richard de Rochemont (1976:302) believe that this cuisine basically was so close to English cooking that it was absorbed almost without notice. The Dutch emphasized abundance and hearty eating. American cooking owes much to the Dutch influence. The common cookie was first a Dutch delicacy, *koekje*. They also produced the "oil cake," crullers, doughnuts, waffles, dumplings, and cole slaw (an adulteration of the original *cool sla*, meaning cabbage salad).

German Cooking

Like Dutch cooking, this cuisine also was very compatible with the new American fare. But, rather than becoming lost within the national cuisine, it became integrated without losing its own identity (Root and de Rochemont 1976:303). German dishes, virtually unmodified, were simply added to the existing American repertory, usually under their original names. Americans consumers have adapted so totally to these foods that they are frequently unaware that their names are actually German words. Examples include sauerkraut, pretzels, pumpernickel, sauerbraten, and wiener Schnitzel (veal cutlet, Vienna style).

Other popular German contributions to American cuisine are apfel strudel, hot potato salad, along with many cheeses and sausages. The Germans gave America its most popular sausage, the frankfurter (sometimes called wiener, or hot dog). Originally, it was a pure beef sausage. However, it has since undergone various modifications, including the use of other types of meat (chicken, pork, mutton, or even goat), changes in fat content, and the use of various extenders.

The Scandinavian Influence

Among ethnic cuisines other than the three just described, Scandinavian cooking perhaps is the most similar to what we think of as American cuisine. Yet, even Scandinavian food is confined chiefly to Scandinavian ethnic enclaves in the United States. When the Scandinavian component becomes high enough within a given region, some of their foods become well enough accepted within the local area that they become regional dishes. Their breads and cookies have been most widely accepted. Examples include Danish pastry, and various coffee breads, such as *julekage* (Christmas cake) and Lucia buns (for the Swedish St. Lucia Day, the festival of lights). The Scandinavians have been given much of the credit for perpetrating the American coffee break and for originating many of the pastries that go with it.

In some areas, particularly in Minnesota, the Dakotas, and Wisconsin, *lefse* is accepted beyond the Scandinavian enclaves. The most widely rejected Scandinavian food is *lutefisk* (literally, "lye-fish," or lye-soaked cod). While the lye treatment served admirably, in earlier days, as a method of preservation (always difficult, at best, with fish), it does nothing for the flavor of the cod. The Scandinavians serve it with large amounts of drawn butter.

The smorgasbord undoubtedly is the greatest of the Scandinavian influences on American eating. The original smorgasbord is immensely popular with Danes, Swedes, and Norwegians alike. It essentially is a buffet-style meal, including both hot and cold dishes. It can consist of as many or as few dishes as the hostess or host wishes, but the overall effect must be appealing and well balanced. Typical foods on an authentic smorgasbord will include fish, meats, and cheeses, a main entree, desserts, and beverages. Herring and beet salad (*sild salat*) and Swedish meatballs are traditional items. This style of eating has long been popular in the Upper Midwest, where many Scandinavians live, not only for meals within the homes but at restaurants and at community affairs. It has since become universally used throughout the United States (and throughout Europe, as well) and usually is referred to as a buffet. It ranges in form from a simple array of appetizers or hors d'oeuvres at a bar or cocktail party to an elaborate buffet supper.

Other Ethnic Cuisines

Although other ethnic cuisines have not entered the mainstream *en bloc*, many individual foods from various ethnic groups have been widely accepted throughout most of the United States. Examples include beef stroganoff (Russian), goulash (Hungarian), borscht (Russian and Polish), various Chinese dishes, and enchiladas and tortillas (Mexican). Certain ethnic dishes which have been converted to a very modified form are considered to be "pop foods" (see below). A well-known example of this is French fries. They seem to have first appeared in the United States in the 1860s and are thought to have been adapted from the *pommes frites* of France.

REGIONAL FOODS

Regional foods are somewhat unique food products or dishes that tend to characterize a particular locality. A strictly regional food would be one which developed within the area. Such foods are, above all, influenced by availability, followed by the ethnic background of settlers in an area. It is understandable that regional dishes tend to reflect strongly those foods which are plentiful in the environment (e.g., fish, shellfish, certain fruits and vegetables). Regional foods are fostered and nurtured by isolation. They are most likely to develop and persist, without significant changes, in small pockets or localities with little contact with the outside world. An example is the Cornish pasty, which still endures in the somewhat isolated regions of the Upper Peninsula of Michigan and northern Minnesota, although the Cornish miners are long since gone.

Regional vs. Indigenous Foods

Regional foods are not synonymous with indigenous foods. Even local plants and animals are often not truly indigenous, having been introduced from elsewhere. When the Indians crossed the Bering Straits into the New World, they still were essentially foragers, with only minimal food procurement techniques, let alone food preparation skills. It seems safe to say that any Asian culture that the Indians may have brought with them had been erased long before they encountered the first Europeans. The skills in food procurement, production, and preparation that they possessed by the time the Conquistadors arrived had to have developed over the millennia since their arrival in the Western Hemisphere from Asia. Thus, strictly speaking, the only truly indigenous dishes in North America were those developed by the American Indians during pre-Columbian times.

Evolution of Regional Foods

The first European explorers and settlers brought their eating habits and preferences with them. In fact, to assure themselves of an ongoing supply of their native foodstuffs and dishes, Columbus and subsequent explorers routinely brought seeds, plants, and animals with them on their sailing vessels, to provide many of the customary ingredients. Thus, to some extent, familiar dishes could be prepared in the new places without change. But many dishes inevitably became modified (and eventually Americanized) by the need to substitute local, available substances for certain customary ingredients. The Indians also exerted a strong influence toward modification, as they showed settlers new techniques and new foods available on the new lands. Later, the dishes were influenced by the arrival of settlers from other ethnic groups, who also made culinary contributions to the cuisine of each area. Examples of this phenomenon abound in the history of America's regional cuisines. The more isolated a group of settlers, the less the cuisine changed because of new food availabilities or new methods of food preparation.

The first contribution to American cuisine unquestionably was that of the native Indians. The Spanish, as the first European explorers and immigrants, exerted the second influence. However, the Spaniards were not true colonizers; their early influence was limited to the southern United States. The Northern European colonists provided a third, and much stronger, influence. The introduction of African laborers into Jamestown, Virginia, in 1619 marked the introduction of yet another dimension. African cuisine has affected the character of U.S. eating habits in many ways, particularly in the South.

Along the Eastern Seaboard, regional dishes developed in the thirteen English colonies, which were strongly characteristic of British and German cooking, since the early colonists were mainly of this ancestry. Early colonial cooking soon became modified by interactions with Indians. Later, it was influenced by African slaves, particularly in the South. In the Southern colonies, a country style of cooking developed, utilizing foods which were raised on the plantations.

In Florida, and along the Gulf Coast, the regional dishes were influenced by Indians, the Spanish, the French, and the Africans. The distinctive Cajun cooking of Louisiana evolved from French, Indian, and African influences, while Creole cuisine derived from all four.

In the Southwest, extending from West Texas to the Pacific Ocean, a different type of cooking developed. It was characterized by dishes originating from both Indian and Spanish standbys, modified by local conditions (Nichols 1959). The influence of Mexican cooking, itself a mixture of Indian and Spanish cuisine, also is evident.

It has been observed that the Midwest and West have few truly regional dishes because they were settled later than these other regions by people from other areas of the United States, who brought their cuisines with them. However, many foreign-born immigrants have come to these areas as well (especially the Midwest). When their numbers have been large enough, some of their dishes have become sufficiently accepted to become regional dishes.

Ethnic versus Regional Dishes

It is to be remembered that an ethnic group must be present in relatively large numbers in order for its dishes to become regional dishes. Otherwise, their ethnic dishes remain "local phenomena." A local (food) phenomenon is a food or dish used almost solely within the homes of the ethnic group or at ethnically sponsored events; it has not, at least yet, become part of the region's general cuisine. An example of an ethnic food that enjoys regional status in one locale and local-phenomenon status in another area, relatively nearby, is that of Belgian trippe (Figure 9.1). Namur, Wisconsin, is the center of the nation's largest settlement of French-speaking Belgian-Americans. This enclave covers an area along Green Bay 20 miles wide and

50 miles long. Within this area, Belgian trippe (a sausage made of lean pork and cooked, chopped cabbage seasoned with nutmeg and other seasonings) definitely is a regional food. In the city of Green Bay, however, some 20 miles from Namur, Belgian trippe can be obtained at a local meat specialty shop. But it is not widely consumed. There, it is considered an ethnic food (a local food phenomenon). By contrast, Polish sausage, another ethnic food, is so commonly consumed in northeast Wisconsin that it deserves regional status (Figure 9.2).

The characteristic regional dishes of general areas within the United States will be described in this chapter within the context of the various influences by which they have been shaped. The states have been grouped into the following seven areas: the Northeast, the South, the Midwest, the Rocky Mountain region, the Southwest (and California), Hawaii, and the Northern Pacific region (Table 9.1).

Northeast

Regional dishes developed in the home kitchens of the early colonists. The dishes that they brought with them from their native lands (mainly England and Germany) were Americanized by the necessity of using locally available food and the influence of friendly Indians (Nichols 1968:357).

From the Indians, the English cooks learned to use corn, not only in breads, but in many cooked dishes, as well as eating it fresh from the cob. Most of the corn dishes which resulted were modified to conform to the familiar tastes of the British Isles. In both New England and the South, those cooks made corn puddings, sometimes as one-dish meals, sometimes to accompany meat, sometimes to finish the meal as a dessert. Both the Indians and the colonial cooks relied on the one-dish meal, which has been used almost universally, throughout history, worldwide. Not only was it compatible with their scanty cooking equipment, it also was a big time-saver, as it is for contemporary cooks.

A well-known dish in the Northeast is dried beans and dried corn cooked together to a porridge-like consistency, called samp. Often cooked with salt pork or pig's knuckles, it is essentially a thick soup or stew.

Succotash is another famous regional dish made of dried beans and corn, but baked or cooked to a casserole consistency. It is a variation of the original *msickguatosh*, introduced by the Narraganset Indians to colonial cooks. There are many so-called authentic ways to make succotash; they may involve the addition of chicken and salt pork, potatoes and turnips, along with the basic ingredients of beans and corn (Jones 1990:9).

Hasty pudding is a Yankee adaptation of an English recipe for an ancient porridge that combined wheat flour, butter, spices, milk, and sometimes an egg. Colonial cooks substituted cornmeal for the wheat flour and, thereafter, often called it Indian pudding. Hasty pudding is still a Yankee fa-

Figure 9.2
Polish Sausage Days, Pulaski, Wisconsin

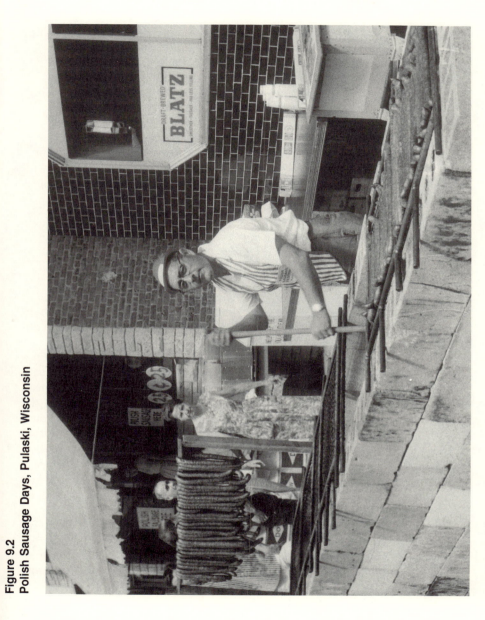

Neville Public Museum of Brown County

Table 9.1
Regions of the United States

Region	States
Northeast	Connecticut, Maine, Massachusetts, New Hampshire, New Jersey, New York, Pennsylvania, Rhode Island, Vermont
South	Alabama, Arkansas, Delaware, Florida, Georgia, Kentucky, Louisiana, Maryland, Mississippi, North Carolina, South Carolina, Tennessee, Virginia, West Virginia
Midwest	Illinois, Indiana, Iowa, Kansas, Michigan, Minnesota, Missouri, Nebraska, North Dakota, Ohio, South Dakota, Wisconsin
Rocky Mountain	Colorado, Idaho, Montana, Nevada, Utah, Wyoming
Southwest	Arizona, New Mexico, Oklahoma, Texas, California
Hawaii	Hawaii
Northern Pacific	Alaska, Oregon, Washington

vorite. There are many variations of hasty pudding (or Indian pudding). In many parts of the country, they often are sweet in flavor and baked in an oven, with accents of maple syrup, molasses, or grated orange (Jones 1990: 10–11).

Other important dishes of the region are Boston baked beans, New England baked bean soup, New England baked beans, Boston brown bread, and "ryaninjun" bread. The latter bread is made of rye flour and cornmeal. Originally, brick ovens were used, which were designed to turn out, at the same time, not only baked beans but bread, Indian puddings, meat pies, and rustic desserts known as pandowdies (16). Red flannel hash is another Down East favorite, made with beets, bacon, potatoes, and onions. Shoo fly pie is a Dutch specialty. Actually, it is a molasses cake, although it is baked in a pie crust. The dessert supposedly derived its name from the fact that flies are attracted to its sweet stickiness, and, continually, must be shooed away (Root and de Rochemont 1976:216–17).

Pennsylvania Dutch scrapple is an aromatic mixture of Indian cornmeal and pork sausage, seasoned with sage and marjoram, formed into a loaf for slicing. It was considered a proper breakfast essential in colonial times. This food still is called Philadelphia scrapple, even though much of it now is made on the farms or in such Pennsylvania Dutch towns as Reading.

Anadama bread is a well-known yeast bread made with flour, a small amount of corneal, and molasses (Jones 1990:208). The generous use of molasses, both in New England and the South, derived from the easy availability of molasses during colonial times, from trade with the West Indies, where it was a by-product of sugar manufacture.

The South

Southern cuisine. The South is known for its style of cooking, which reflects the foods that traditionally were produced in abundance on its plantations.

Typical foods include corn dishes, rice, ham, barbecued ribs, yams and sweet potatoes, red eye gravy, greens, hominy (including grits), and hog 'n' hominy. The latter is a special combination of salt pork and corn often credited with keeping pioneers alive in every phase of western migration. Ashes and water convert corn to hulled, dried corn in the making of hominy, "a Southern fetish" (Jones 1990:8). Hominy, when coarsely ground, is known as grits; another gift from the Indians, it is one of the most characteristic foods of the South. It can be served as a gruel, with maple syrup (Jones 1990). Red eye gravy contains small pieces of ham and probably originated in poor homes, where meat was scarce. It now is a typical item on a southern menu, especially in restaurants catering to tourists.

Other favorites are peanut soup (Virginia) and catfish (fixed various ways). Then there are desserts from oranges: ambrosia, a southern dessert, and orange pie, popular in Virginia and other parts of the South. In the South today, chicken wings in barbecue sauce are popular in bars and restaurants, and bourbon is generously used in cooking: bourbon pie, steaks marinated in bourbon and spices. Barbecued foods (again, barbacoa) reflect both Indian and Spanish influences; the Spanish first learned the techniques from the Indians, and they later added the spices (Jones 1990: 73). The southerners' love of spices reflect both the Spanish and African-American influences.

Breads include spoon bread, corn pone (corn bread made without milk or eggs), corn sticks, johnny ("Jonny") cake, and hush puppies, all originating with the Indians. Spoon bread (or batter bread) has been a southern favorite since colonial times. During the twentieth century, it has served as a common substitute for mashed potatoes in the South.

Popular African-American (soul) foods include greens, black eyed peas, corn pone, hominy, pork ribs and backbones, hocks and chitterlings (small intestines of the hog) (Ferguson 1989).

Creole cooking. Creole cooking originated along the Gulf of Mexico, and its dishes are still considered to be characteristic of this region extending from West Florida through Brownsville, Texas. However, New Orleans and Louisiana's River Road plantations are considered the home of the distinctive cuisine most often described as Creole cooking (Jones 1990:48). The term "creole" comes from the Spanish word *criolla*, which means "native to the place," especially with respect to Spanish Americans. Creole food can be viewed as a true melting pot, having developed from early, highly flavored Spanish dishes, modified by the Indians, and later, by African slaves, who were being brought to New Orleans by the 1700s. After Louisiana became a French colony, the delicate foods of the French were integrated into this unique cuisine, which have been described as "cheerfully unconscious of Anglo-Saxon cooking" (Root and de Rochemont 1976: 281). The word "creole" is often used to identify spicy concoctions often dominated by green pepper, onions, and garlic.

New Orleans cuisine reflects numerous cosmopolitan influences. It was a center of trade, receiving foods from South and Central America via the West Indies. In addition, exotic spices and foods were introduced to New Orleans by travelers returning from Mexico.

Foods which are particularly representative of Creole cooking are rice, beans (including red haricot beans), chorizo (Spanish sausage referred to as *chaurisse* by the French descendants of Louisiana), andouille sausage, and jambalaya.

Jambalaya perhaps is the most distinctive Creole dish. It derives its name from having been made originally with ham (*jambon*). Rice is the foundation for this dish, to which seafood, ham (and sometimes other meat) and tomatoes are added. A classic New Orleans recipe combines shellfish with spicy Spanish sausage (chorizo), country ham, highly seasoned pork link sausages, and tomatoes, along with cayenne pepper.

Cajun cooking. This cuisine is associated with the Acadians, deported French Canadians who settled in the bayou country, west and south of New Orleans, after 1755. Essentially, it is country food, reminiscent of its ancient French origins, further modified by the influence of Louisiana Indians and slaves. Original Cajun cuisine was not influenced by the Spanish; it also had little of New Orleans or Paris. However, in later years, there has been some blurring of the boundaries between Cajun and Creole cooking.

Typical Cajun dishes include gumbo, crawfish dishes, and boudin sausage. Gumbo is a type of bouillabaisse, or fish stew. A bouillabaisse, by itself, is not unique, since every country which has access to fish makes fish stews, or thickened fish chowders. But "gumbos" are special thickened chowders to which either okra (an African contribution) or filé (dried sassafras powder, an Indian contribution) is added as a thickener. Only Louisiana has discovered the gumbos; and the New Orleans version is unique: it is a special hybrid creation, since both okra and filé are used.

The Cajun boudin sausage is of two types: boudin blanc and boudin rouge. The boudin rouge (red sausage) is a spicy blood pudding, and it is in danger of no longer being available commercially because current regulations for livestock-slaughter inspection make the collection of blood difficult and unprofitable (Sokolov 1981:8). White boudin is made with a pork and rice stuffing. It is a loose sausage, fiery and pale colored, with a strong taste of liver and kidney. The sausage (moderately warmed by steaming) is eaten by holding the casing in one's hands and sucking the insides from the casing (125–26). It would appear that, although the future of boudin rouge may be threatened, the outlook for boudin blanc seems to be promising, if the annual Louisiana Boudin Festival held in Broussard is any indication. At this event, young men and women may be observed competing in a boudin-eating contest, "slurping stupendous quantities of pork and rice stuffing out of long, drooping casings" (26).

The base for Cajun stews and gravies is the *roux,* a mixture of flour and fat. However, the Cajun roux is unique in that the flour and fat (usually vegetable oil) are heated very slowly, until the mixture turns brown and has a nutty taste.

Other key ingredients in Cajun cooking are rice, which has been grown in Louisiana since the early 1700s, red beans, tomatoes, chayote squash, eggplant, spicy hot sauce, and a variety of pork products. One of the better-known hot sauces, Tabasco, is produced in the bayous of southern Louisiana from fermented chili peppers, vinegar, and spices. A deep-fried rice fritter, *calas,* is the Louisiana version of a doughnut. Other rice dishes are red beans and rice and "dirty rice." Dirty rice is so called because two of its ingredients, bits of chicken gizzards and liver, give the rice a brown appearance.

Louisianans often flavor their coffee with their indigenous chicory root. Pecan pralines are a famous New Orleans candy. Pecans are native to Louisiana; pralines are large flat patties made from brown sugar, water or cream, and butter. Another confection eaten often with coffee are *beignets,* round or square puffed French doughnuts dusted with powdered sugar. French toast, or *pain perdu,* is another French specialty that was transported to New Orleans and is now familiar to most Americans. A famous Louisiana dessert is a frothy cooked orange cream made with orange juice, sugar, eggs, rich milk, and the accent of lemon.

Creole cooking is to Cajun cooking what French *grande cuisine* is to provincial, or French country, cooking. Ingredients in both Creole and Cajun cooking reflect the abundance of fish and shellfish in the Louisiana environment. Catfish is popular in foods ranging from Creole to soul food to pop food.

Florida cuisine. In the Southeast and in Florida, particularly, the Continental Spanish influence, modified by the produce of tropical islands, has resulted in the distinctive cuisine known as Creole, along the rim of the Gulf of Mexico (Jones 1990:59–60).

The conquistadors introduced black beans into Florida from their Caribbean islands, along with more exotic ingredients, such as the orange. In Tampa, rice is mixed with black beans to make a "sobering" dish for midnight suppers at late parties (for example, on New Year's Eve). Ponce de Leon, early in the sixteenth century, brought rum to the mainland from the

Caribbean, where it was used to point up the oregano and garlic flavor of baked black beans.

The influence of its island neighbors is reflected in many Florida dishes. Examples are pigeon peas with rice Puerto Rican style, *arroz con pollo*, and *arroz con carne* (rice with chicken or beef). Chick peas, or garbanzos, were introduced by the conquistadors to the developing cuisine of the area.

Typical dishes of Florida and the Keys include *bolichi*—eye of beef stuffed with a mixture of piquant Cuban-style sausage, pimiento-stuffed olives, green pepper, onions and other vegetables, with accents of lime juice and cumin seed. Both of the latter are Spanish influences. Other dishes are *alcoporado*, a beef stew, with raisins to offset the piquancy of its other flavors; and *piccadillo*, a mixture of minced beef, raisins, and olives, usually served with rice. Florida is one of the leading commercial fishing states in the United States, and its plentiful fish resources are reflected in its cooking. Shrimp, lobster, scallops, crabs, pompano, and red snapper are readily available. Evan Jones describes snapper fillets served in a common Floridian style with a Spanish sauce, or as snapper fillets baked with orange rind, a soupçon of juice, and seasoned with pepper and nutmeg (Jones 1990:64).

Florida is the leading avocado state. It also produces many other exotic fruits. Orange desserts are popular, as well as desserts from chayote squash (accented by raisins and rum, topped with an almond-sprinkled meringue) (Jones 1990:72).

The Southwest and California

Oklahoma. The rolling plain of Oklahoma, before the advent of the whites, was originally covered by herds of buffalo and populated by roving Indians who followed them as their source of livelihood: food, clothing, and shelter.

The land turned out to be well-suited for agriculture. Beef, dairy products, chickens, and hogs are the chief sources of income. Leading crops are wheat, sorghum, and many kinds of fruit (including cherries, berries, persimmons, and peaches). There also are walnuts, pecans, and hickory nuts, along with some game and fish. An offbeat specialty that Oklahoma shares with Texas is mung beans, grown for the food industry, which converts them into sprouts.

Texas. This state has a variety of soils and climates, as well as areas of mountains, timberland, farmland, range and pasture, and a rich coastal plain with a subtropical climate.

Mainly, the colonists entered Texas from the Northeast and spread to the south and west. In these areas, there were herds of wild horses and cattle, survivors from animals brought by the early Spanish conquistadors. To the north of the early colonized area, the plains were still the realm of the buffalo (first reported in 1541) (Root and de Rochemont 1976:46).

Texas Longhorns descended from these wild cattle. More beefy, palatable breeds have long since been introduced.

The early colonists wanted to plant corn, the indispensable grain of the pioneer. It became very important to the Texas pioneers: fresh corn, porridge, corn breads, cornmeal, corn "molasses" for sweetening. There was no shortage of meat (much of it game), on Texas tables, in the first half of the nineteenth century.

Because of the wide variety of environments in Texas, regional food differences developed early. On the Gulf, for example, there is an abundance of oysters and other seafoods. In addition to cotton, the Coastal plains grow many garden vegetables, including corn and sweet potatoes. In the southern border cities, especially, Mexican dishes early began to be popular. Beef and game traditionally have been plentiful.

The hallmark of Texas cooking is the barbecue. Texans pride themselves on their preference and tolerance for strong flavors and spices. For example, East Texas boasts of its spicy specialty sausage, known as "Texas hot guts." Texans are known for their pecan ice cream and candy ice cream.

Texas has more deer than any other state (followed by Michigan). It also has pronghorn and wild turkeys, mountain lions, and wild pigs (javelina). It is a leading agricultural state, in large part because of irrigation. Beef cattle provide 50 percent of the farm income. Texas is a leading state in shrimp production. Texas waters also yield blackdrum, crabs, flounder, red snapper, red drum, and sea trout. Farm-raised catfish is another important crop, as is rice, which is grown along the coast. Truck farming (vegetables, fruit, including citrus, watermelon, peaches) also is an important enterprise in Texas.

Arizona. Since irrigation is essential for agriculture in this state, the scarcity of water has enabled only a modest amount of farming. The state produces cattle, dairy products, dates, barley, wheat and other grains, sorghum, potatoes, grapefruit, oranges, lettuce, walnuts, and cherries. The state also grows vitis vinifera (as does California, Washington, Oregon, and Arizona), a species of grape which grows only west of the Rockies. All of these states produce small quantities of very drinkable wine. It also is one of the four chief grapefruit growers, along with Florida, California, and Texas. Available game include the Mexican javelina, the only native pig of North America.

There are many people of Mexican ancestry in Arizona, especially in the southern part of the state; 6 percent of its residents are Indian.

New Mexico. Despite its dry climate, agriculture is this state's fifth source of income. Grazing is the chief form of farming: cattle, dairy products, and sheep head its exports. Sorghum (drought resistant), corn, and beans for drying are other chief crops, but some fruits and vegetables are grown in the Rio Grande and other river valleys. New Mexico has more water than Arizona.

Most New Mexicans are descended from one of the three major groups that settled in the area: Indians, Spaniards, and English-speaking Americans. The Spanish influence shows strongly in place names, foods, and holiday customs.

California. This state has been included with the Southwest region because it shares a common Spanish heritage, and similarities in climate and foods, with those states. To a large extent, irrigation has overcome the problem of limited rainfall, with respect to the growing of many common food products (e.g., the avocado and citrus fruits). Eighty percent of the lemons consumed in the United States are grown in California; it is second to Florida in avocados. It is one of the leading states in commercial fishing, which yields a wide variety of seafoods, including shellfish. Tuna is the most valuable seafood product, followed by crab.

California has a varied cuisine, which includes Tex-Mex foods and mainstream American food, along with dishes which are more pristinely Spanish. The Mexican influence is to be expected, since Mexicans make up the largest group of foreign-born residents. *Menudo*, which has both Indian and Spanish origins, is eaten here. San Francisco Bay is the home of *yerba buena*—"good herb," which grew wild over the hills above the bay and added a special flavor to the cooking of meat and other foods in the early period. Some modern California cooks substitute tarragon mixed with chervil or parsley to give a gentler flavor. Lamb here is often seasoned with juniper berries (preferably the wild ones). Safflower blossoms are used as flavoring, as well as piñon (pine) nuts, and olives. A dish developed in the Sierras is fresh perch flavored with almonds, pine nuts, and olives. Pheasant is made with chorizo (Spanish sausage); turkey *mole* (pieces of turkey in a Mexican sauce of dried chilis, chocolate, and many other seasonings) is popular. Together with poultry and pumpkin seed sauce, and gazpacho Pasadena, they are representative of the many California dishes with both Spanish and Indian nuances. The plentiful orange is used in salads and desserts (including ambrosia, which is also popular in the South). Spanish green olives, usually stuffed with pimiento, are a California contribution to American eating habits (Jones 1990:79). Dishes with a Spanish origin include roast pork infused with oregano and garlic, covered by thick brown sauce containing accents of ripe native olives, chopped green pepper, and tomatoes.

Many Californians of Chinese and Japanese ancestry live in enclaves in Los Angeles and San Francisco. They, along with more recent immigrants from Southeast Asia and elsewhere, have also contributed ethnic influences to the culinary scene. Sourdough bread, so important to California's pioneers during the Gold Rush days of the mid-1800s, is still baked today.

Tex-Mex food. The term "Tex-Mex food" refers to a particular kind of American cooking found along the Mexican border of Texas, New Mexico, Arizona, and California. It is American food strongly influenced by Mexican cuisine; therefore, it has both Spanish and Aztec elements. As the name implies, Texas claims credit for it, probably because its shared border with Mexico is longer and more populous than that of the other three border states. (This food is not synonymous with the commercial types of Mexican food that have found their way into supermarkets and fast-food establishments across the country, i.e., pop food).

The Spanish sausage chorizo is used in Tex-Mex cooking. Chili powder is generously used, especially in the making of chili con carne and chili con arroz.

Tex-Mex food in Texas is very highly spiced, in keeping with the general penchant of Texans for strong flavors. The Tex-Mex food of Arizona is more closely related to authentic Mexican cooking than that of Texas. However, the tortillas are made of wheat flour rather than the usual corn tortilla of most of Mexico. The Arizona food also is much less highly spiced, using milder chilis, than prevailing Mexican cuisine. *Menudo,* the earlier-mentioned soup made from tripe and hominy, is borrowed from Sonora and is served in Arizona. Tex-Mex food is more widespread in New Mexico than Arizona, because it still has many descendants of the old families of the Mexican era. They call themselves Spanish-Americans and maintain the culinary traditions of the past, including many dishes which are more Spanish than American. Examples include a special anise-flavored Christmas cookie, little hot breads called *sopaipillas,* which are served with a sauce containing cinnamon (a favorite spice of Spain). Cinnamon also is used in *caperotoda,* Spanish bread pudding. The baked pudding *panocha* is a genuine Indian dessert of Aztec origin, made from sprouted wheat. However, the Spanish now have modified it with a dash of cinnamon, also.

The Rocky Mountain Region

In addition to being geographically contiguous, the Rocky Mountain states share other characteristics. Lack of rainfall presents a problem in growing food crops in the Rocky Mountain area. Fortunately, Colorado, Idaho, and, to some extent, Nevada, have access to water from rivers and lake(s) within their borders. Nevada's agriculture is minimal, and what there is depends on irrigation. Lack of water forces Montana, Wyoming, and Utah to rely heavily on dry farming and grazing for the production of wheat, cattle, and sheep. Colorado and Idaho utilize dry farming and grazing as well.

The regional dishes can be described as basically "all-American," since the original settlers came primarily from the East and Midwest, and an overwhelming percentage of the current residents were born in the United States. As to be expected, those food crops, fish, and game which are abundantly available locally inevitably play an important role in the regional cuisines.

All of these states are landlocked. Therefore, seafoods must come in from outside the area. However, the Rocky Mountain states are noted for their many kinds of fresh-water fish. The cold, swift streams of Montana, Wyoming, and Idaho are especially known for various kinds of trout. Both Montana and Idaho produce salmon. Nevada has the distinction of producing a fish called *cui-ui*, a large sucker found only in Pyramid Lake. It was once an important food fish among the local Indians. Mutton is produced from sheep by Basque herdsmen who were brought from Spain to the Mountain States toward the end of the nineteenth century.

The Rocky Mountain region is still wild enough that it is good game country. Buffalo meat, which resembles choice roast beef in flavor, is becoming a Western specialty. There now are two sources of buffalo meat: government-protected herds and domesticated bison raised by private breeders. States in the area which are producing bison include Montana, Wyoming, and Utah. Both game animals and game birds are plentiful in the region.

In Winnemucca, Nevada, there is Basque-style dining in restaurants, and oven-roasted mutton, or even mutton hash, are fixtures on the menus. Jones states, "Basque cooking is straightforward and filling, with few frills—not even simple desserts" (Jones 1990:75).

Nevada, Idaho, and Wyoming raise most of the area's sheep. Cattle raising is economically important to Idaho, Montana, and Wyoming. Idaho is noted for its famous Idaho potato, which is superb for baking, and it also grows appreciable amounts of apples, peaches, pears, cherries, and plums (for prunes). Hops is raised for beer in Idaho, along with its sister states, Washington and Oregon.

Wyoming's Starr Valley boasts an unexpected specialty from a state that has never had many milk cows—a type of cheese similar to Swiss Emmenthal, from 5,000 Holstein cattle in the valley—⅛ of all the cows in the state. It is made by Mormon families who settled there before 1900.

Wyoming families consider trout as traditional for the Christmas holidays as turkey or ham in other parts of the country. Fish is usually frozen in blocks of ice and when cooked, it has that fresh-from-a-cold-stream taste.

Since 70 percent of Utah's residents are Mormons, it is not surprising that they have had a tremendous influence on the state's food habits. Because of the early years of want in Utah, the Mormons are highly motivated to possess a secure food supply. Each family keeps underground stores of wheat and other staples. Mormon cooking emphasizes quantity rather than quality; foods are bland. The drinking of tea, coffee, and alcoholic beverages is discouraged. Without caffeine, the universal American stimulant, the Mormons appear to turn instead to sweets. Their consumption of sugar is very high, particularly in the form of candy and baked goods.

"Game cuisine." All of the Rocky Mountain states can be said to be

"venison country," and cooks in the area have developed considerable expertise in fixing this meat. They insist that venison is superior to any other kind of meat for both mincemeat and chili con carne. Some natives insist that game is best when served with red currant jelly or currant jelly mixed with horseradish. Quince and grape jellies are considered good game accompaniments, too.

The Pacific Northwest

Along with Idaho, the land that is now Washington and Oregon originally was part of "Oregon Country." Oregon became a state in 1859; Washington joined the union in 1889. Both states share the Columbia River, which serves as their dividing boundary. Thus, the two states share a common source of fish, shellfish, and crustaceans. Both have concentrated on the development of orchard fruits, for which the climate seems to be eminently suited. Washington and Oregon are noted for their numerous distinctive fruit pies and cobblers. They also share a small specialty called "firewood honey"—gathered from a plant which grows profusely after forest fires. Along with Idaho, they grow hops for beer. Both states are known for special cheeses: Washington for its Cougar Gold and Oregon for its Tillamook (cheddar) cheese.

Washington is well known for its Dungeness crab (also available from Alaskan waters), considered by some to be the tastiest in America. Washington's chief income from seafood comes from salmon, especially chinook and sockeye, then from oysters and crabs. Other distinctive seafoods are the Olympian oyster, which comes from Puget Sound; the Pacific oyster, a very large oyster imported from Japan in 1902, clams, and pink shrimp. Both states have rainbow trout, as do many of the Rocky Mountain states; this fish originated in the West.

Agriculturally, Washington is best known for its fruits, especially apples. Wanatchee Valley is the chief apple-producing region—growing mostly the Delicious and Winesap varieties. In addition to apples, Yakima Valley grows pears, melons, and grapes and makes some wine.

Numerous Swedes in the state have added ethnic interest to local cuisines, especially with their Swedish coffee bread and Swedish cakes and cookies (Root and de Rochemont 1976:310).

Oregon's first commercial fruit was the apple, followed by the pear—which became the pride and glory of Oregon. The Hood and Rogue River valleys are famed pear-producing regions of the Northwest. The state also is important for its berries, plums, and sweet cherries. In fact, a popular intermediate-price restaurant chain offers Oregon Berry Shortcake Supreme as a regular dessert item. Dungeness crabs and salmon are the most valuable fishery products.

Some Oregonians trace their ancestry back to the Oregon Trail. The largest groups of foreign-born are from Canada, Germany, Great Britain, and Mexico.

Alaska. Fish is the chief source of both food and revenue in this state. Salmon (especially chinook and sockeye) is the major seafood product, but the product most readily associated with Alaska is the huge Alaskan king crab. Alaska also is known for Dungeness crab and the snow crab.

Alaskans are called "sourdoughs," because, in early pioneer days in Alaska, it was essential to have a "starter" for bread. Keeping a homemade starter going was a universal need for pioneers, when commercial yeast was not available, because bread was such an essential staple. Although commercial yeast is now available to most Alaskans, many still pride themselves on keeping sourdough (some of which is as old as 50 years). Homemade bread is still a prized food staple.

The native population consists of Indians, Eskimos, and Aleuts. Some Eskimos still eat whale. They often rely on a fish diet, supplemented in summer by berries and roots, plus caribou. They are especially fond of the cloudberry, one of the best sources of vitamin C.

Next to the caribou, moose is the most important game. An Alaskan specialty is moose meat, prepared in thin, dried slices. Another delicacy is the Alaskan Dall sheep, whose meat tastes like spiced young lamb. Berries and mushrooms also are important regional foods (Root and de Rochemont 1976:266).

Hawaii

The 1959 addition of Hawaii as the fiftieth of the United States marked the addition of a number of new, exotic foods that contribute an exotic dimension to American cuisine.

Only 15 percent of the inhabitants of Hawaii today are genuine Hawaiian, i.e., descendants of the original Polynesians who began to arrive on the Hawaiian Islands around A.D. 750. Their food originally was seafood. Later, their diet was supplemented by fruit, which arrived on the islands by various routes and grew well. There also were no cereals in Hawaii when the Polynesians arrived. The chief cereal there today, and the only one really suited to growing conditions, is rice. The sugar industry began in 1835, and pineapple raising began early in the twentieth century. Macadamia nuts, which originated in Australia, were first planted in Hawaii a century ago. Now the islands have a monopoly on the commercial production of these nuts.

The coconut palm has played an important role in shaping Hawaiian eating patterns. The juice pressed from the meat is used instead of cow's milk for many things. For example, it was used as a sweetener before the arrival of sugarcane. The coconut also provides palm hearts—the terminal buds of the coconut palm—which is a favorite vegetable. The sap of the palm can be processed into wine, spirits, or vinegar.

Pigs were brought by Polynesians from Southeast Asia and are still the favorite meat of Hawaiians. Chickens have been in Hawaii a long time and are a well-accepted food.

During the nineteenth century, Hawaiian cuisine included many diverse foods, a reflection of the diverse peoples who had come to develop Hawaii. They included New England missionaries, Chinese plantation owners, Japanese sugarcane workers, Koreans, Portugese, and some Scots (Steinberg 1970). However, as more and more missionaries arrived during the growth of the sugarcane and pineapple industries in the late 1800s, eating habits changed dramatically. At the present time, the most commonly consumed food is that of the mainland United States. Hawaiian supermarkets carry the usual U.S. products and brands, plus Hawaiian foods which have been Americanized.

Fortunately, the fish and fruits of the region have endured from the early days. Turtle and Kona crab and Kona coffee are additional food delights. The latter two products are raised on the west side of the island of Hawaii.

Traditional Hawaiian cuisine is most visible when luaus are held (often for tourists). Luau originally meant taro, but now it means feast. In the making of *laulau*, chopped taro leaves are added to leaf-wrapped packages of steamed food such as fish and pork or fish and chicken. (Hawaiians often combine meat with fish.) Poi is the pounded root of the taro, from which a starchy paste is made and served from a bowl. Everyone eats from this bowl, without silverware, by dipping in with the fingers. A sort of punch, with or without rum, is served throughout the feast (Hawkins and Hawkins 1976:274).

The centerpiece of a luau is the pig, cooked in a pit (*imu*), with the aid of heated stones. The animal is stuffed with stones and cooked from both inside and without, so thoroughly that the flesh tends to fall apart upon serving. Other foods are steamed at the same time, wrapped in leaves. *Ti* leaves, which impart a musky flavor, are used for fish. *Limu*, an edible seaweed, also is steamed.

Distinctive Hawaiian food specialties are *pipikaula* (jerked beef broiled in tiny pieces and served with a sweet-sour sauce), *lomi lomi* (thin fillets of salted salmon, mixed with chopped onions and tomatoes and served as salad), and appetizers such as *pupus* (chunks of pineapple broiled in a wrapping of bacon or cubes of barbecued pork) and *rumaki* (bacon-wrapped kebabs of chicken livers and water chestnuts). Many of these foods have found their way to the mainland, particularly California (Jones 1990:167–68).

The Midwest Region

Often called the Central Plains Region, this vast 12-state area consists generally of flat land. It is especially suited to agriculture, although irrigation is needed in some areas. The region's farms produce great quantities of corn, wheat, and other crops, livestock, and livestock products. The Midwest also produces large quantities of fruit.

The area is blessed with the Mississippi River and its tributaries, the Great Lakes, and other smaller lakes, rivers, and streams. Almost all of the states boast good recreational fishing opportunities. Some states, particularly in the Great Lakes Region, also have commercial fishing industries. In addition, large amounts of large game and game birds are available in many areas. All of these assets make for an abundance of food in this region.

In most of the Midwestern states, 96 percent or more of the residents were born in the United States. Many of them have descended from residents of other states who moved to the region. But there also are large groups who are descendants of settlers from Europe. Foreign-born residents include those from Canada, Germany, Great Britain, Hungary, Poland, Italy, Yugoslavia, the Netherlands, and the various Russian republics. More recently there are increasing numbers from Southeast Asia. Most of these groups have contributed ethnic foods to the areas where they have settled.

It has been said that the Midwest has few truly regional dishes, because it was settled originally by people from other parts of the United States who brought their local dishes with them. Another factor that has undeniably had a "homogenizing" effect on Midwest cuisine is one which is evidenced throughout the United States. It is the easy availability of mainstream and "pop" foods in restaurants, fast-food places, and supermarkets.

However, regional foods do exist, though unfortunately, space does not permit an exhaustive listing. One example is Bess Truman's Ozark pudding, a favorite of President Harry S Truman of Missouri and his wife (Jones 1990:481). It is a simple custard pudding, containing chopped apple, chopped walnuts, and rum and is served with whipped cream. The Great Lakes area is the scene of many seasonal "trout boils" (Figure 9.3), where trout and boiled potatoes, both swimming in melted butter, are enjoyed. Smelt is a popular food in Michigan, Minnesota, and Wisconsin. Here, each spring, smelt buffs eagerly await the arrival of spawning smelt, as they travel from Lakes Michigan, Huron, and Superior up local streams and rivers. At this point, they can be caught easily with either hooks or nets (Figure 2.3). Despite their small size, those who like smelt seem more than willing to assume the arduous task of preparing the large numbers needed to make a family meal.

North Dakota is noted for its chokecherries, high bush cranberries, and wild plums. South Dakota also has chokecherries and wild currants. Wisconsin has blueberries, huckleberries, Juneberries, wild black currants, and cranberries; Wisconsin's Door County is noted for its apples and cherries. Honey is an important by-product of the fruit industry, especially in Central Michigan.

Figure 9.3
Supervising the Fish Boil at Trout Festival, Kewaunee, Wisconsin

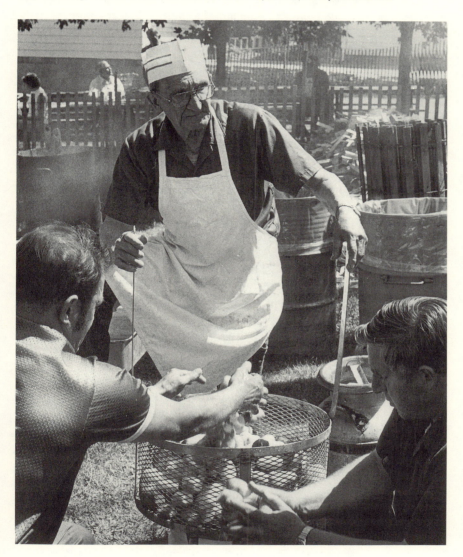

Neville Public Museum of Brown County

POP FOODS

"Pop" foods include fast food, "food on the run," and foods with an ethnic "twist" that have become commercialized and Americanized enough that they usually are significantly different from their authentic ethnic origins. Fast foods (see chapter 6) include hamburgers, cheeseburgers, fishburgers, French fries, pizzas, and various types of Mexican foods (e.g., tortillas, tostados, tacos, and burritos). These foods can be obtained not only at fast-food restaurants but in the frozen food sections of grocery stores. Some fast foods are more regional in nature, reflecting local foods. For example, oysters and catfish (e.g., catfish sandwiches) are important pop foods in Alabama. And, in New England, along the Atlantic, lobster rolls (served warm, with a side order of onion rings) have been available at roadside eateries for generations. Another traditional fast food of the Northeast is breaded clams fried in deep fat.

Some pop foods with an ethnic twist are processed and distributed universally throughout the United States in food stores. Common examples include Chinese-influenced foods (e.g., chow mein and chow mein noodles) and Italian-like foods (e.g., canned spaghetti, macaroni, ravioli, and Spaghetti-O's, usually with a tomato sauce base).

Food on the run refers to small snacks eaten before going to work (or school) or during lunch breaks, usually from on-site vending machines or at short-order places. These include coffee, juice, fruit, rolls, and other snack foods. This food behavior is becoming increasingly common in America today.

Pop food may lack creativity and, in many cases, it suffers from dietary faults shared by much of America's contemporary cuisine: too much salt, fat, or sugar. Nevertheless, the future of pop food seems assured. It is convenient, usually less expensive than most other prepared foods, and represents a saving in time for the busy traveler, businessperson, or homemaker—who may be juggling the demands of home and family with a full-time job. Many Americans have become so accustomed to the taste of pop food products that they actually prefer them to most home-cooked dishes.

FOR FURTHER READING

Ferguson, S. 1989. *Soul food.* New York: Grove Press.

Hall, R.L. 1991. *Savoring Africa in the New World.* In H.J. Viola and C. Margolis, *Seeds of change* (161–69). Washington: Smithsonian Institution Press.

Hawkins, N., and A. Hawkins. 1976. *The American regional cookbook.* Englewood Cliffs, NJ: Prentice Hall.

Jones, E. 1990. *American food* (rev.). Woodstock, NY: Overlook Press.

Kittler, P., and K. Sucher. 1989. *Food and culture in America*. New York: Van Nostrand Reinhold.

Pamela, P. 1969. *Soul food cookbook*. Bergenfield, NJ: New American Library.

Root, W., and R. de Rochemont. 1976. *Eating in America*. New York: Ecco Press.

Sokolov, R. 1981. *The fading feast*. New York: Farrar, Straus, and Giroux, Inc.

Figure 10.1
Plants Engineered to Stay Healthy

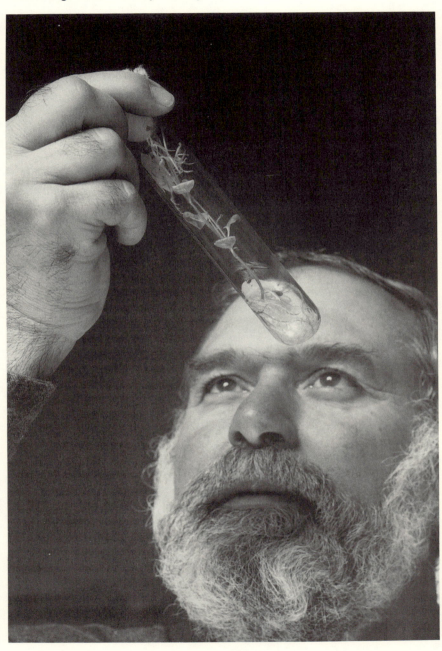

Plant pathologist examines a tissue-cultured potato plantlet genetically engineered with anti-bacterial genes. Agricultural Research Service, USDA.

The American Diet: An Assessment and Prognosis

Over time, the North American diet has evolved through stages that are strikingly similar to those experienced by other societies today considered technologically advanced. Roughly speaking, all of these societies have obtained their food first by foraging, followed by hunting and collecting stages; then rudimentary forms of food production (horticulture and animal husbandry) have followed. The latter then have evolved into intensive agriculture and other forms of food production and, finally, to large-scale mechanized agriculture, including both plant and animal production. With these changes have come periodic fluctuations in dietary adequacy. Now these countries are moving into the postindustrial stage of biotechnology, which will bring further changes in dietary adequacy.

Throughout history, the most powerful influence on human eating habits and choices has been the factor of availability, since one cannot eat what one does not have. Availability, in turn, is influenced by geography, climate, economic status, politics, and other factors (chapter 7).

In assessing the American diet over time, one is forced to make generalizations. Generalities, unfortunately, are difficult and can be misleading, because of the diversity of population groups existing within each time period. There always are groups within a given time frame who have widely different food availabilities, either in quantity or quality, for one or more of the reasons cited previously. Therefore, this assessment, of necessity, will focus on representative eating habits for each period. Certain health statistics are closely linked to nutrition and provide objective information that is helpful in making nutritional assessments. They include mortality rates (especially infant mortality), morbidity rates (certain diseases are especially nutrition sensitive), life expectancy at birth, as well as stature and growth trends. Where available, such information will be used in making these nutritional assessments.

DIETARY TRENDS AND NUTRITIONAL ASSESSMENT

The Pre-Columbian Period

Early foragers. The history of American food begins with the North American Indians, who descended from Asians. They are thought to have crossed the Bering Straits from Siberia at least 20,000 years ago, as the fourth Pleistocene glaciation receded. These people were food foragers who searched for plant and animal foods without the aid of special techniques. Thus far, they had discovered neither tools nor agriculture. It is believed that they and their descendants, the Paleo-Indians (13000–8000 B.C.), continued to use this most rudimentary method of obtaining food for several thousand years.

Upon arriving in what is now Alaska, these Asian immigrants undoubtedly depended mainly on animal food, supplementing their diet with the few plant foods that were available in this subarctic area.

How adequate was the diet of these foragers? The absolute quality of their diet probably was fairly good, since they did eat animal foods. The most reliable source of nutrition for animals is the flesh of other animals, particularly when the entire animal is consumed. It is known, for example, that various animal organs are high in vitamins A and C, as well as the B vitamins. In addition, if they lived near the ocean, seaweed would have provided additional high amounts of carotene (vitamin A). Also, cloudberries, in season, would have been another rich source of vitamin C.

Milk was not part of their diet, since they had no domestic milk-giving animals. Their calcium intake, largely from fish and animal bones, plus a small amount from plant sources, probably was marginally adequate.

Although their diet probably was reasonably well balanced, undoubtedly it often was inadequate in amount. Because of the limited technology for obtaining what already constituted an uncertain food supply, life must have been precarious. As is true even for the present-day Eskimo, both birth rates and death rates undoubtedly were high, and the life expectancy low.

Paleo-Indian Period (13000–8000 B.C.). By 10000 B.C. or before, the descendants of the immigrant foragers had become hunter-collectors who had learned to make tools and missile weapons. These instruments enabled them to obtain vastly more meat in the form of the large animals that were roaming the grasslands during this pre-Boreal period. They also could collect plant foods more efficiently. These advances obviously made for a better, more dependable food supply. As long as food was reasonably plentiful, this diverse diet should have been nutritionally balanced and adequate.

The Paleolithic Indian is thought to have consumed about 5 pounds of food a day, consisting of about 35 percent meat (mostly game) (1 ¾ pounds), and 65 percent plant foods (3 ¼ pounds). This diet is believed to have provided about 3,000 Kcalories a day. It was high in protein and complex carbohydrate, but relatively low in fat, since most of the meat was consumed as game. Although this diet was high in complex carbohydrates, it was low in concentrated sweets. The only sugar consumed was obtained from fruits and an occasional treasure trove of honey, upon discovering a bee hive. The high intake of plant foods would have provided a large amount of fiber, probably about 45 grams daily (Eaton and Konner 1985).

Archaic Indian Period (8000–1500 B.C.). At the beginning of this period, the Indians were continuing to practice both hunting and collecting, that is, obtaining both animal and plant foods using special techniques. Nutritional adequacy would have been generally good. Later, however, there were new shifts in climatic conditions. The grasslands dwindled, and oak and hickory forests began to cover large areas.

The disappearing grasslands, upon which the large animals depended for sustenance, led to a sharp reduction in their numbers, which, in turn, led to overkilling. These two circumstances, together, eventually led to their extinction. The Indians now were forced to hunt smaller animals for meat, providing much lesser quantities. Fortunately, the new Boreal climate favored the growth of plants, upon which, through necessity, the Indians now became increasingly dependent for their daily diet. As a result, collecting, as a food-getting activity, was stimulated. Conditions now were favorable for the development of horticulture, which is thought to have emerged in North America during this epoch. According to Claire Cassidy's studies, the protein intake and general quality of the diet of hunter-gatherers during this period was high (Cassidy 1980:129).

Woodland Indian Period (1500 B.C.–A.D. 300). Horticulture led to the real beginning of agriculture (albeit on a small scale) during this epoch. "The emergence of the hoe provides technological evidence that plants were domesticated during this period" (Jerome 1981:38). With greater consumption of plant foods and less animal food, diets now were high in complex carbohydrates and much lower in protein. These early agriculturists also were consuming more potassium and less sodium than when animal foods constituted the dietary staple. Consequently, they are thought to have suffered often from salt hunger—the need for more sodium. This need was fulfilled by exploiting more and more smaller animals and eggs, as well as fish and desiccated sea water, when available in the environment.

Mississippian Indian Period (A.D. 300–1500). By the time Europeans began to arrive, the North American Indians had diffused both southward and eastward, into Central and South America, the Caribbean, and to Eastern North America. At the time of Columbus's landfall, the Indians, both in the West Indies and on the North American mainland, were well into the latter part of the Mississippian Period. This period is marked by the beginnings of intensive agriculture (or at least advanced horticulture; see chapter 3). Staple crops were corn, beans, pumpkins, and squash. In addition to agriculture, hunting and fishing remained important (Jerome 1981:38). Wild fruits, roots, and berries lent variety to this diet. The diet was nutritionally adequate as long as the supply of these diverse food resources was sufficient. However, as the focus on agriculture increased, less time and energy were available for hunting, fishing, and collecting. As result, the variety of the diet decreased, with adverse nutritional consequences. Moreover, with agriculture came increased population densities, with more competition for the existing animal and plant foods in the environment. As a result, the diets of agriculturists, who were relying mainly on cultivated corn, beans, and squash, with only modest supplementation with wild animals and plants, became high in complex carbohydrate and relatively low in protein.

Consumption of alcohol. In all early cultures, alcohol consumption has come about initially through naturally occurring fermentations of sugar-containing fluids, from foods in the environment (fruits and other plant juices, honey, and the milk of mammals). Since fermentation requires a reasonably warm temperature, it is unlikely that the earliest North American foragers, who were living in what is now Alaska, had much access to alcoholic beverages. Thousands of years later, as the Indians dispersed to warmer latitudes, they undoubtedly discovered fermented juices, first by accident. Later, they learned to make them, deliberately. Records of North American Indians drinking alcohol, particularly in the more temperate zones, are sparse. When the Europeans arrived, they introduced the Indians to their distilled (hard) liquors, such as West Indian rum (Root and de Rochemont 1976:83).

Nutrition-linked health statistics. Claire Cassidy attempted to assess the nutritional impact of agriculture on pre-Columbian Native Americans by studying the skeletal remains of two precontact village sites in Kentucky. The older village, Indian Knoll, had been inhabited by foragers (hunter-collectors) about 5,000 years ago during the Archaic period, while Hardin Village had been inhabited by agriculturists about 1,000 years ago (during the Woodland Indian era). Cassidy found that the hunter-collectors had life expectancies at birth of 22 for males and 18 for females (associated with a high infant mortality rate, which rose to a maximum life expectancy at ages 2 to 4 of 27 for males and 23 for females). The agriculturalists had a life expectancy at birth of 17 for males and 18 for females, reaching a maximum life expectancy at ages 5 to 6 of 21 for females and 19 for males. At Indian Knoll, 44.6 percent of the children died before age 17, while at

Hardin Village, the corresponding figure was 53.7 percent (p <0.05). At Indian Knoll, 70 percent of mortality under age four [4] occurred in the first year while 60 percent of infant and toddler mortality at Hardin Village occurred between ages 1 through 3 (p <0.001). The latter circumstance is indicative of protein calorie malnutrition (Cassidy 1980).

According to John Verano and Douglas Ubelaker (1991:215), considerable morbidity existed in the pre-Columbian New World, because of a number of diseases, particularly respiratory diseases, dysentery, tuberculosis, and perhaps treponemal disease (syphilis). The result was a high mortality rate and reduced life expectancy. These authors state that in some regions, mortality, especially infant mortality, was increasing through time, presumably in response to increased infectious disease resulting from more crowded and less sanitary living conditions. However, since these vital statistics are very much influenced by nutrition, it can be assumed that malnutrition also was an important factor (Scrimshaw, Taylor, and Gordon 1968).

"Several well-controlled demographic reconstructions from archaeologically recovered samples suggest that life expectancy at birth for aboriginal populations in the New World was between 20 and 25 years, reflecting high rates of infant mortality. Adult age at death averaged in the mid-thirties. Figures for different times and places varied considerably, but they are quite similar to those estimated or recorded for European cities during comparable periods" (Verano and Ubelaker 1992:215).

The Colonial Period

The foremost nutritional problem facing the earliest European settlers in North America was adequate food. Undernutrition, malnutrition, famine, and starvation were frequent threats (see chapter 4). The story would have been much grimmer had it not been for the help from neighboring Indians. Miriam Lowenberg and her associates (1979) have observed that once the colonists (with the help of the Indians) learned what food was available and how to get it and cook it, the supply was plentiful. In fact, the colonists were better supplied with food than any other people in the world at that time.

Very soon, the colonists were duplicating the bland English cooking to which they were accustomed, now modified and embellished with new Indian accents. By today's standards, their Anglo-American cuisine would be perceived as monotonous and unimaginative, with its overwhelming heaviness and sparse use of spices. The colonists used sweetness, particularly after 1750, both in desserts and other dishes, to counter this blandness (Levenstein 1988:6). In fact, after 1750, Americans and Britons possessed the Atlantic world's greatest sweet tooth, with Americans running a close second to Englishmen in per capita sugar consumption (Mintz 1985:188).

Corn was the basic cereal, followed by rye. Both were used in making rye 'n' Injun bread (1:1). Wheat did not mature well in New England, so little was used.

One of the main deficiencies of early Anglo-American cooking was its lack of fresh vegetables and fruits. Few vegetables were used, not because they were unavailable, but because, like their British counterparts, the colonists were accustomed to using vegetables primarily in sauces or garnishes, to accompany the meat dish.

While no nutritional surveys were carried out during this period, the diets had to have been lacking in certain vitamins and minerals as a result. Milk consumption probably was low; meat, especially pork, probably was adequate for most. The colonial diet, generally, was high in fat, salt, and sugar. The pork was consumed mainly as salt pork, since salt served as an excellent and readily available preservative.

Consumption of alcohol. By the time that colonists began arriving in America, all Europeans who could afford it were drinking large amounts of alcoholic beverages, because the water was not dependable. The early American settlers were heavy drinkers, too, for basically the same reason, at least initially. However, even British visitors to the colonies were astonished by the amount of liquor Americans drank (Root and de Rochemont 1976:356), presumably an indication that their consumption of alcohol considerably surpassed that of the British. The early white settlers were well acquainted with the production and use of alcoholic beverages, both fermented and distilled.

Nutrition-linked health statistics. Most of the colonists were shorter than Americans are today. Judging by the subsequent overall rise in stature in America, from colonial times up to the present, the diets of early settlers must have been limiting, at least with respect to certain key nutrients. By today's standards, the health of the colonists was poor (Martin 1989a: 4, 798). Most people suffered frequently from various illnesses, which they did not know how to treat or prevent. There was a scarcity of doctors and nurses during the colonial period. Despite this poor medical care, it probably was no worse than that of Europeans during this time (Martin 1989a). From all indications, low life expectancies, high death rates, high birth rates and high infant mortality rates were the rule during colonial times. Nevertheless, during the Colonial Period in America, European health statistics were worse (Verano and Ubelaker 1991:223).

In 1789, at the end of the Revolutionary War, life expectancy was 34.5 years for men and 36.5 for women (perhaps largely a reflection of high infant and child mortality rates). Sexagenerians in 1789 could look forward to 14.8 more years of life (Cummings 1970: Appendix C). In the late eighteenth century, the mean stature of Americans almost reached modern levels. By the time of the American Revolution, native-born white males aged 24 to 35 measured 68.1 inches, which is virtually identical with heights in the

U.S. Army during World War II (Fogel, Engerman, and Trussel 1982:415–16). The fact that this value for height was comparable to modern levels would suggest a fairly high level of nutrition. However, it is not known whether these men (presumably soldiers) were representative of the general population. From the fact that European males during the late seventeenth and early eighteenth centuries were 2 to 4 inches shorter than 68 inches (15), it seems certain that first generation colonists from Europe during that period generally were of similarly short stature.

Although the final height of African-American males at the end of the eighteenth century was an inch less than that of native-born whites, they were 1 to 3 inches taller than blacks born in the Caribbean and Africa (Fogel, Engerman, and Trussel 1982:416). These data for blacks indicate that, despite the hardships of slavery, African Americans were experiencing better living conditions (particularly nutrition), than counterparts in their countries of origin.

The Nineteenth Century

The earlier years. In the light of current nutritional knowledge, many persons within both the rural and urban sector suffered from serious dietary deficiencies during the period 1789–1850, the early years of the republic. The rural staples were corn and potatoes, along with pork, bread, and butter. Hogs and hominy were mainstays throughout most of America and despite their limitations made survival possible over much of this period. Nevertheless, throughout the country, consumption of the perishable foods—milk, fresh fruits and vegetables, as well as fresh meats—was inadequate. Urban workers and their families were less well fed than the rural population because they could raise little if any of their own food and had limited resources with which to buy what foods were available in the city at this time. The lack of fruits and vegetables, and subsequently lowered fiber intake, undoubtedly contributed to the constipation chronically experienced by Americans during this period, both in the rural and urban sectors. Lack of fruits and vegetables, as well as milk, also led to the lack of numerous vitamins and minerals necessary for proper growth and maintenance of the body. These included vitamin C, riboflavin, and calcium, as well as vitamins A and D. Many people probably were suffering from lack of vitamin C, unless they were eating substantial amounts of potatoes and cabbage. According to Everett Dick (1937:275), some of the pioneer children on the western plains suffered from scurvy from lack of vitamins (undoubtedly vitamin C, and others).

Unless large amounts of butter and cheese were consumed as a substitute, the customary low milk intake could have resulted in both vitamin A and D deficiencies. It is known that rickets was a common problem among infants and children. Lack of milk and leafy green vegetables undoubtedly resulted in suboptimal intakes of calcium for many; inevitably this would contribute to reduced growth and stature. Americans were generally smaller in stature than they are today. Lack of elements found in milk also may have contributed to the decayed, spotty, and missing teeth of both young and old (Volney 1804:226–27; Mesick 1922:90). Because of the low consumption of milk and leafy green vegetables, riboflavin deficiency must have been common. Lack of this vitamin can cause eye problems ranging from sore, running eyes to cataract formation as well as various types of skin lesions.

Vitamins and minerals also are associated with the body's defense toward disease (particularly vitamin C, vitamin A, and zinc). The lack of many of these nutrients must certainly have been an important factor in the prevalence of disease, especially in the cities, during this period.

Along with dietary lacks, there also were dietary excesses. Intakes of both fat and salt were high, according to Volney (1804:323). Particularly on the farms, people had access to large amounts of butter, fatty cheese, lard, and salted pork products, including hams and sausages. Salt provided a practical, much needed means of preserving pork. However, despite the practice of soaking salt meat products before use, salt consumption still was too high. This salty diet also may have encouraged the excessive use of sweeteners, since they were thought to "cut the salt," or mask its flavor. (Unfortunately, the relationship between salt and high blood pressure was not recognized by the medical community until the 1940s.)

A pattern of high intakes of sugar, fat, and salt had developed in the South, because of the ease of obtaining molasses (and later, sugar) from the West Indies and the large amount of pork raised and preserved with salt on the plantations. This pattern still continues today.

Obesity appears not to have been a problem during this period, despite the high fat intake of many. The most likely explanation is that most people had a relatively moderate total caloric intake, coupled with a high activity level (particularly on farms). Thus, excess calories (from fat or other sources) would have been burned off as energy.

The later years. During the latter half of the nineteenth century, dietary improvements occurred in the rural population. In general, rural people were consuming more milk, fruits, and vegetables, and beef. However, hogs 'n' hominy remained critical for survival in those southern and western communities who still were without rail service (Cummings 1970:86). According to Frederick Law Olmsted, southern planters generally subsisted on bacon, sometimes cooked with turnip greens, corn pone, and coffee sweetened with molasses instead of sugar (Olmsted 1860:396). It must be remembered that single croppers usually considered it economically unwise to invest labor and land resources for growing food crops, with the exception of corn.

The lot of city workers generally was better during the latter part of the nineteenth century. Their buying power had improved. By the 1850s and 1860s, they were buying and consuming more lean meat, milk, leafy vegetables, and fruit. But although milk consumption had increased, its mean per capita consumption was only ⅓ of a pint (Cummings 1970:77), an amount still substantially below today's recommendation of one pint or more daily for adults. By the late nineteenth century, the nation's total nutrition had improved (Atwater 1887). However, according to Wilbur Atwater, many Americans were eating far too much with respect to both total food (energy) and nutrients (meat, fats, and sweetmeats) (Atwater 1888b:262).

Whereas constipation was the nation's curse of the first half of the nineteenth century, dyspepsia became the prime digestive complaint of the mid- and late nineteenth century, especially of the upper middle class and aristocrat groups (Levenstein 1988:22). These largely urban individuals were particularly prone to overeating, partaking of heavy, greasy, sweet, and generally difficult-to-digest foods and a considerable amount of alcohol. This was particularly true of men. However, women also were consuming more food than is customary today. Dyspepsia and overweight were common among both women and men. However, the degree of overweight was more pronounced among men, who displayed their abdomens with pride, as badges of their prosperity (12).

Overweight does not seem to have been a concern among the city workers, for whom getting enough food still was the major challenge. Neither constipation nor dyspepsia seems to have been a problem with them, judging from the lack of complaints voiced in this regard. Since whole grain meals were cheaper than refined white flours, they consumed mainly whole grain rather than white bread. It may have been to their advantage that their diets were coarser and contained more fiber. Immigrant families of this period also consumed fair amounts of vegetables; they raised gardens and were likely to engage in home canning.

Consumption of alcohol. According to Waverly Root and Richard de Rochemont (1976:377), "The drinking habits of the early nineteenth century were excessive." By 1825, the per capita consumption of alcoholic beverages in terms of total absolute alcohol was 3.7 gallons (Rorabaugh 1979:232). Thereafter, old-stock Protestants turned increasingly against liquor (Grover 1987:28). Their diminished use of alcoholic beverages was partially offset for a time by the substantial consumption of alcohol by newly arriving immigrants and the continued drinking of the upper class. But by 1840 net per capita consumption of alcohol had plummeted to 1.8 gallons (expressed as absolute alcohol). Alcohol use declined further during the remainder of the century (Rorabaugh 1979:272). According to W.J. Rorabaugh, middle-class drinking habits underwent a profound change between the end of the Civil War and the beginning of the twentieth century. Beer displaced whiskey and other hard liquors, and the trend toward abstinence (which became associated with respectability and propriety) increased (20).

Rorabaugh believes that the underlying reason for the "robust drinking" of the early nineteenth century was the unprecedented change that occurred between 1790 and 1830. He has noted that during this time "almost every aspect of American life underwent alteration, in many cases startling upheaval. . . . and . . . those groups most severely affected by change were also the groups most given to heavy drinking" (125).

Overall nutritional status. Despite the failings of the American diet during this period, the nutrition of Americans, if not ideal, was substantially improved. The intake of milk, as well as fruits, vegetables, and beef had increased. Their better total nutrition is saliently demonstrated by their increase in both size and girth, longer life expectancy, and other positive changes in health statistics.

Nutrition-linked health statistics. The mean stature of Americans almost reached modern levels in the late eighteenth century, indicating that the United States enjoyed a relatively high nutritional status at that time. But around 1830 mean stature of Americans began a prolonged decline, which continued until at least the 1870s. This mean decrease in height is thought to be a reflection of the poor condition of many members of the working class (Fogel, Engelman, and Trussell 1982:415–17). Generally, they were shorter than more affluent Americans (Gould 1869:295). The industrialization and urbanization of the first half of the nineteenth century produced not only an affluent and expanding middle class but also an era of inequality and poorer nutrition for American workers (Lindhert and Williamson 1976).

At greatest risk were the children of city wage earners. A survey of pupils in the public schools of Boston in 1875 revealed that, as a whole, they were better developed than children in English schools, but those who came from the families of laborers were inferior in physique to those from more prosperous families (Bowditch 1877:297–98, 307).

Gordon Bowles (1932:30–31) observed that the stature of Harvard men had been increasing for at least 80 years (i.e., since approximately 1852). He considered this increase to have been fastest shortly after the Civil War. By the 1880s, Americans had increased in both size and girth to the point that manufacturers of ready-to-wear clothing (geared mainly toward the middle class) were forced to adopt a larger scale of sizes. These gains in body size are a strong indicator of better total nutrition, at least among middle-class Americans (Cummings 1970:89).

Robert Higgs (1975:177–95) calculated that from 1880 to 1930, rural death rates declined by 30 to 40 percent. He ascribed this "vital revolution" mainly to better diet.

Edward Meeker (1972:353) estimated that "average mortality and life expectancy improved little, and likely worsened, prior to 1880," but that "a fundamental transition in the state of health occurred in the decade of the eighties." There were improvements in both life expectancy and mortality, brought about primarily by improved nutrition. Sexagenerians who might have looked forward to 14.8 more years of earthly existence in 1789 had an expectancy of 15.6 years a century later (Cummings, 1970:88 and Appendix C—commenting on the calculations of Edgar Sydenstricker, a noted public health statistician). According to Grace Peckham, the life expectancy of infants at birth had increased from 34.5 years in 1789 to 41.7 years in 1880. But many were ill fed; it is estimated that the infant mortality rate was twice as high in the city as in the country (Peckham 1885:82–84).

Overall infant mortality rates from 1850 until the end of the century were at least as high as those of the developing world today. They varied from 123/M in 1855 to a peak in 1870 of 170/M (U.S. Department of Commerce, Bureau of the Census 1976). The latter figure is similar to those for the poorest Third World countries today.

Infant death rates for African Americans were even higher. Throughout the nineteenth century, they ranged from 266 to 278 per thousand for males and 222 to 237 for females. Mean life expectancy for African Americans during the nineteenth century was about 33.7 years for both sexes (Eblen 1974:301–19). It is of note that these shocking vital statistics are strikingly similar to those for the general populace in Europe during the later nineteenth century (Richardson 1887; Defnet, Ducat, Eggericks, and Poulain 1986).

The Twentieth Century

During this century, much more quantitative information has become available regarding the eating habits of Americans. Thus, a more definitive assessment of food consumption patterns can be made for this period than has been possible for previous eras in American history.

Longitudinal trends in food consumption. During the last century, per capita consumption of animal products in the United States increased in relation to crop products (including flour and cereal products), but not dramatically. According to Ben Senauer, Elaine Asp, and Jean Kinsey (1991:14), a saturation level, not only of animal products, but of total food, has been reached by affluent societies like the United States. As a result, the food consumption stabilizes. Total per capita food consumption has actually declined in the United States since 1945, with the largest share taken out of crop products. The energy content of the food supply has been remarkably stable during the century. In 1987, 3,500 Kcalories per day were available in the food supply, compared with 3,400 in 1910, and a low of 3,100 in 1957 (Hiemstra 1968; Putnam 1989).

After a generally downward trend in the consumption of meat, poultry, and fish between 1910 and 1935, there has been a spectacular rise during the remainder of the century in the consumption of these items. Pork consumption has been quite stable throughout the century. There has been a spectacular rise in the consumption of poultry since the mid–1930s. In 1989, on a boneless, trimmed weight basis, per capita poultry consumption was 4.5 pounds less than beef and 18 pounds more than pork. Poultry consumption soon may surpass that of beef. Pork consumption surpassed beef until the mid-1950s, when the latter increased markedly after 1950 until the late 1970s. Since then, the general pattern of beef consumption has been one of decline. Fish consumption has been remarkably stable over the century, increasing slightly since the early 1980s. In 1989, it still represented only 8.3 percent of the total meat, poultry, and fish consumption (Senauer, Asp, and Kinsey 1991).

There has been a spectacular rise in the consumption of eggs (after the mid-1930s), followed by a dramatic fall after the mid-1950s. The consumption of dairy products also fell, with a moderate rise in the 1980s due mostly to cheese consumption. There appears to be a significant relationship between health concerns about fat and cholesterol and these decreases in consumption of milk, beef, pork, and eggs (Smith, Herrman, and Warland 1990).

Over the century, Americans have steadily increased their overall consumption of fat while substituting vegetable for animal fat. Essentially, the consumption of animal fat has declined since 1940, and the consumption of vegetable oils has increased steadily since 1909, overtaking animal fats in 1950.

There was a substantial drop in the consumption of flour and cereal products, from 300 pounds per capita in 1909 to 172 pounds per capita in 1988 (Hiemstra 1968; Putnam 1989; Putnam 1990). In recent years, however, there have been increases in the consumption of cereals and grain (Smith and Yonkers 1990, Putnam 1991). According to Judith Putnam, the average per capita consumption of wheat flour rose 24 percent from 1970–74 to 1990, when it reached 138 pounds. An important factor in this rise is that Americans are eating more pizza, pasta, pitas, and fajitas, all of which are made from wheat flour. There also has been increased consumption of breakfast cereals, particularly those containing oat bran. This trend is attributed to the public desire for more fiber. Although fiber intake has increased markedly since the late 1970s, it is still well below the recommendation of the National Cancer Institute of between 20 and 30 grams per day (Butrum, Clifford, and Lanza 1988).

The per capita consumption of fresh fruits has declined from 123 pounds in 1909 to 94 pounds in 1988 (Hiemstra 1968; Putnam 1989; 1990). Although fresh fruit consumption has increased since 1970, it still is less than was consumed before 1950. These trends can be explained in part by the demise of home-grown and home-processed fruit during the first half of the century. Apples, bananas, and citrus have remained the dominant fruits over the century.

There has been a steady increase in vegetable consumption since 1909. Total fresh vegetable consumption has increased 42 percent since 1970 alone. As with fruits, the most common reason given for increasing fresh vegetable consumption are concerns about health and nutrition (United Fresh Fruit and Vegetable Association 1988). Although overall vegetable consumption has increased over the century, there has been a large decline in potato consumption (73 percent of all vegetables in 1909 versus only 30 percent in 1987). Part of this decline undoubtedly can be attributed to the increased popularity of pasta and other wheat products. For example, per capita consumption of pasta products rose from 9 pounds in 1970–74 to 13 pounds in 1990. Even so, potatoes, along with iceberg lettuce, are the two most popular vegetables in America. In 1990, they constituted 37 percent and 17 percent of fresh vegetable consumption, respectively (Liebman 1990).

There has been a phenomenal increase in the use of all types of sweeteners. Per capita consumption now exceeds 150 pounds per capita. This trend has occurred, despite a decline in the consumption of refined cane and beet sugar since 1972, because the use of corn sweeteners and noncaloric sweeteners has increased substantially. It is ironic that despite the use of artificial sweeteners, Americans are consuming more sugar than ever before. The rise in total sweeteners is connected with the rise in the consumption of soft drinks, almost all of which are now sweetened with either corn sweeteners or a noncaloric sweetener (Senauer, Asp, and Kinsey 1991: 28).

Coffee consumption peaked in 1946 at 20 pounds per capita, then fell back to a little more than 9 pounds in 1977 (its level in 1914). Subsequently, it has risen and is currently holding steady at about 10 to 11 pounds per capita (Hiemstra 1968; Putnam 1989). The use of decaffeinated coffee and specialty gourmet coffees has increased. Because of price competition, many large coffee companies in the United States have been using the cheaper robusta bean (which produces a mild-tasting coffee), rather than the high-grade arabic bean. However, consumers who have discovered the gourmet blends now prefer them (Robichaux 1989).

The consumption of alcohol has decreased significantly. During the early part of the twentieth century, drinking still was heavy, at least among urban workers. Beer had become the alcoholic beverage of choice by the end of the early 1900s. A minute minority drank wine (Root and de Rochemont 1976).

After prohibition laws became effective on January 16, 1920, the drinking of alcoholic beverages dropped sharply. Then, with the repeal of the 18th Amendment in 1934, the drinking of alcohol increased, particularly among the prosperous. By 1990, although alcohol consumption in the

United States was decreasing, about 9 percent of the total population were consuming more than two beverages daily (USDHHS/PHS 1990). During the forty-year period from 1949 to 1989, general whiskey consumption decreased from 80 percent to 38 percent of all spirits consumed. Vodka consumption rose from 1 percent to almost 24 percent of hard liquor consumption. Sales of beer and wine also have increased greatly since 1949. The jump in popularity of beer and wine may be explained by consumers' desire for beverages with a lower alcohol content. John Farquharson, president of the National Restaurant Association, has predicted that alcohol consumption probably will never revert to the per capita levels of earlier decades (Dustan 1991:A6). Americans currently are drinking much less than at any time since the beginning of the century, with the possible exception of the prohibition period.

Compliance with dietary recommendations. How well are Americans complying with the Dietary Guidelines of 1990? Ironically, from calculations based on gross consumption data of Senauer, Asp, and Kinsey (1990: 13–31), Americans were doing better in 1909 than at any time since, including today. Consuming 43 percent of their diet as complex carbohydrate, 11 percent as concentrated sweets, about 30 percent as fats, and about 16 percent as protein, they were (inadvertently) following the Guidelines quite closely.

Complex carbohydrate consumption decreased to about 30 percent in 1940, and to 24 percent in 1960. Although in recent years, some health-conscious Americans are eating more complex carbohydrates in the form of pasta, grains, and potatoes, mean per capita consumption of complex carbohydrates still has risen only slightly since 1960. On the other hand, the consumption of sweeteners had risen significantly by 1940 and has continued to rise. In spite of the consumption of noncaloric sweeteners, we are eating more sugar and corn sweeteners than ever before. Salt consumption, although presumably lower than during the first three centuries of United States history, is still generally higher than the Guidelines recommend. Americans continue to consume far more fat than the 30 percent or less of total caloric intake which is recommended. Despite the many health hazards attributed to excessive fat consumption, most Americans seem reluctant to forgo foods high in fat.

Nutritional adequacy. During the twentieth century, Americans generally have eaten sufficient amounts of total food, calories, and protein. However, after 1909, the general trend has been one of overconsumption of fats, sugar, and corn sweeteners and underconsumption of complex carbohydrates.

Overweight is a common problem. Yet, as pointed out early in this chapter, the caloric intake of Americans has been remarkably stable throughout the century. Therefore, the nation's problem with overweight generally is not due to overeating per se. Rather, it is due to lessened physical activity, which results in less calorie need than earlier in the century, in order to maintain energy balance. Therefore, Americans should be consuming fewer calories (e.g., food that is less calorie-dense), or exercising more, or both.

Since about 1940, there has been a marked rise in the so-called chronic diseases of civilization: hypertension, cardiovascular disease, obesity, and diabetes. It is becoming increasingly evident that these conditions may be more closely associated with diet and exercise than they are an inevitable result of aging.

Despite a tendency toward overnutrition, the diets of many Americans are low in one or more vitamins and minerals, often because of unwise food choices. Common nutrient deficiencies are calcium, iron, and vitamin C.

Nutrition-linked health statistics. Despite its faults, the overall quality of the American diet has improved during the twentieth century, as evidenced by positive changes in certain health statistics that are closely linked to nutrition.

Since 1900, there have been remarkable gains in life expectancy and declines in infant mortality. "They were achieved not only by treatment and by curative medicine, but also by preventive and health-promoting measures, such as improved sanitation, better nutrition, pasteurization of milk, and control of infectious disease" (Owen and Frankle 1986:15).

Robert Higgs (1975) has reported a decline in rural death rates of 30 to 40 percent between 1880 and 1920, which he attributes mainly to better diet. S.L.N. Rao, who views the nineteenth century as having been a period of slow improvement in mortality rates, sees an acceleration of the process in the first half of this century (1973:405, 407). Since 1950, there has been a slower but continuing increase in life expectancy, for nonwhites as well as for whites. In 1900, the life expectancies for whites and nonwhites were 47.6 and 33.0, respectively, versus 76.5 and 71.8 years, in 1992 (World Almanac 1994). This life expectancy figure of 71.8 for nonwhites is almost identical to that for whites (72.0) in 1971, little more than a score of years earlier. During this period, the discrepancy between life expectancies for nonwhites versus whites has narrowed dramatically, a reflection of improving living conditions for nonwhites, particularly nutrition. A large percentage of the twentieth-century increases in life expectancy at birth has come as a result of a great decline in infant mortality rate, which has long been recognized as a gross indicator of the health and nutritional status of a community.

By 1900 Americans were well fed by international standards of that time. Nevertheless, in 1900, America's overall Infant Mortality Rate was 141 per 1,000 (U.S. Department of Commerce, Bureau of the Census 1976). Although lower than that of Europe at that time, this figure is greater than that of many developing countries today. Except for occasional small fluctuations, a continuous decline in Infant Mortality Rate has occurred in this country. The decline was particularly marked after about 1915, the very period when the diets of a large number of Americans seem to have improved (Levenstein 1988:195). By midcentury, the relationship between rising income and lower infant mortality rates held only for those in the lower third of income levels, where an inadequate diet could well be the result of insufficient purchasing power (McMahon 1974:193–95). Overall rates for infant mortality (all races) ranged from 141 in 1900 to 9.2 (per 1,000 births) in 1992 (7.6 for whites and 18.0 for nonwhites) (World Almanac 1994:956).

Visible evidence for improved nutritional status—increased height (and weight)—has been accruing during the twentieth century, continuing a trend that began in the 1880s. Children are becoming taller and heavier and are maturing earlier. The growth in stature of Americans born between 1906 and 1931 was more rapid than that of any other period for which comparable data exist (Bowles 1932:108, 132–33). Collectively, these nutrition-related statistics point to important improvements in nutritional status during the twentieth century.

DIETARY HABITS: WHAT'S AHEAD?

General Trends

For the remainder of the century, salient factors that will influence the American food system include demographic trends, recent dietary recommendations from governmental and professional agencies, and a continuing emphasis on health promotion and disease prevention. Demographic trends, such as the aging of the population, the increase in single-family households, the rising proportions of women working outside the home, the booming ethnic population, and the shift in income distribution, will bring changes in food patterns, creating new food markets. There will be a greater demand for convenience foods. At the Eighth Annual Midwest Food Processing Conference, Gilbert Leveille predicted that fresh or prepared foods that can be microwaved will be the mainstay of future meals. He pointed out that the frozen dinner and entree category (already a proven success) is projected to increase 48 percent by the year 2000 to a $715 billion market (Leveille 1990).

Snack foods and fast foods appear to be here to stay. There is a trade-off in the use of these foods between price and taste and the saving of labor and time. But many busy Americans (including homemakers working outside the home) obviously are willing to make that trade. It is predicted that the nutritional quality of these foods will continue to improve in response to pressure exerted on the food industry by health-conscious Americans.

New nutrition labels evolving from the new Nutrition Labeling and Education Act (Food and Drug Administration 1990) will provide added assistance to consumers as they attempt to follow current dietary recommendations related to diet and health (see Table 6.3, chapter 6). As more Americans attempt to translate these guidelines into daily personal eating patterns, there will be increasing demands for more healthful food products of all kinds. There is a large and growing market for replacements for such macronutrients as fat, sugar, and sodium.

Nouvelle cuisine. Translated literally from the French, this phrase means "new cooking" (Sokolov 1991). Some of the best traits of this postmodern cuisine (discussed in chapter 6), including its simplicity and honesty in food preparation and presentation, will continue. Not only will its influence be observable in the cuisine of upper-scale eating establishments; increasingly, it will permeate mainstream cuisine.

Regional cooking. Regional cuisine will gain strength as the United States matures and Americans become more secure and aware of their national and local identities and the intrinsic worth of our nation's culinary beginnings.

Biotechnology. The twentieth-century revolution—biotechnology—will continue to touch many spheres of our life. It will play a key role in our future food system. Scientists predict that novel biotechnologies will be used in the future (many of them by the end of the 1990s) to change the way many foods are produced and processed. These innovations will have important implications for the consumer. Plant biotechnologists already have developed transgenic plants with improved characteristics (Table 10.1). Biotechnology offers hope as a means of enabling food production to keep pace with the expanding world population and projected food needs.

The trend toward increased use of fresh ingredients and foods will continue, enhancing the opportunity for applying hydroponic systems and biotechnology to provide freshness (Bolaffi and Lulay 1989:266).

Other Predictions

There will be a continued trend toward more upper-scale fast-food places. Much of our food will continue to come from industrial sources and corporations. However, specialty foods still will be available from the smaller independent producer at a higher price.

There will be a continued widespread interest in culinary excellence, reflective of increased travel and sophistication, on the part of Americans. There will continue to be a two-tiered approach to cooking by many homemakers, using fast and convenience foods when expedient, but also engaging in more creative but time-consuming food preparations when time permits. Homemakers will continue their interest in home gardening, canning and freezing, and baking, at least some of the time. At the same time, there will be more meals eaten outside the home, at restaurants and fast-

Figure 10.2
New Varieties of Fruits and Vegetables Produced by Biotechnology

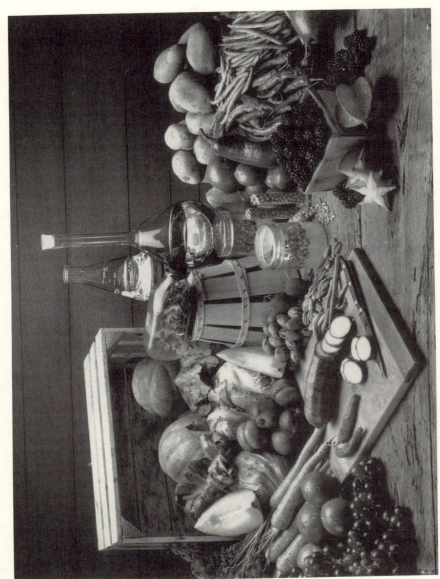

Agricultural Research Service, USDA

Table 10.1
Some Species in Which Transgenic Plants Have Been Developed

Asparagus	Lettuce	Rice
Cabbage	Lotus	Soybean
Carrot	Pear	Sugar beet
Celery	Peas	Sunflower
Corn	Potato	Tomato
Cucumber	Rape	Walnut

Source: U.S. Congress, Office of Technology Assessment 1992.

food places, but also light breakfast/lunch, "grazing" meals at quick-lunch places or from vending machines at or near the workplace.

There will continue to be wide diversity in the diet, though the Anglo-Saxon core will continue. As a result of the consumer movement that began in the 1970s, the American public is more powerful than ever in shaping the products produced by the food industry.

THE AMERICAN DIET TODAY

Melting Pot or Smorgasbord?

The American diet of the late twentieth century is, on the one hand, highly standardized and homogenized, yet also very diverse, reflective of the "new civilization" itself (Toffler 1980). The prediction that the United States, populated by individuals of many geographic and ethnic origins, would one day become a diffuse sociocultural melting pot has not materialized. With unexpected tenacity, the various ethnic and racial groups in America have managed to retain their individuality, including their characteristic food patterns. Admittedly, the uniquely ethnic foods may be reserved primarily for Sundays and special occasions. But they persist (along with more typically "American cuisine"), serving to remind partakers of a common heritage and to provide specific groups with a powerful means of maintaining their identity and cohesiveness.

In addition to the presence of ethnic foods, there still are pervasive regional influences. Further adding to this heterogeneity is the wide availability of snack foods and other pop foods.

At first glance, the diversity of the contemporary American diet may appear chaotic. Yet, on closer scrutiny, a "core" diet becomes discernible, which has its origins in early United States history. The typical dishes which comprise this "baseline diet" reflect British and northern European cuisines—eating patterns brought to America by the early immigrants.

Some order emerges from the initially confusing American culinary scene if one likens it to a large, heavily laden smorgasbord. In the center are the basic dishes of the core diet so familiar to Americans: potatoes of various types, a wide selection of meats, poultry, and fish, various vegetables and fruits, and desserts. On the periphery, as side dishes, are a large selection of ethnic, vegetarian, and regional foods (usually representative of the locale). Snack foods and typical fast foods probably will not be there, but all participants in this feast know that they are readily available at the nearest supermarket or drive-in restaurant.

The overwhelming message that this tempting array conveys is that which has epitomized American foodways since colonial times: an emphasis on ABUNDANCE. This emphasis stems from that compelling motivation shared by most of the immigrants who have come to America over the years—the quest for a secure food supply.

FOR FURTHER READING

Cassidy, C.M. 1980. Nutrition and health in agriculturists and hunter-gatherers. In N.W. Jerome, R.F. Kandel, and G.H. Pelto (eds.), *Nutritional anthropology* (117–45). Pleasantville, NY: Redgrave Publishing Company.

Cummings, R.O. 1970. *The American and his food* (rev.). New York: Arno Press.

Fogel, R.W., S.L. Engerman, and J. Trussell. 1982. Exploring the uses of data on height. *Social Science History* 6(4):401–21.

McMahon, B. 1974. Infant mortality in the United States. In C.L. Erhardt and J. Berlin (eds.), *Mortality and morbidity in the United States* (189–209). Cambridge, MA: Harvard University Press.

Meeker, E. 1972. The improving health of the United States, 1850–1915. *Explorations in Economic History* 9(3):353–73.

Rao, S.L.N. 1973. On long-term trends in the United States, 1850–1968. *Demography* 10(3):405–19.

Rorabaugh, W.J. 1979. *The alcoholic republic.* New York: Oxford University Press.

Senauer, B., E. Asp, and J. Kinsey. 1991. *Food trends and the changing consumer.* St. Paul: Eagan Press.

Verano, J.W., and D.H. Ubelaker. 1991. Health and disease in the pre-Columbian world. In H.J. Viola and C. Margolis (eds.), *Seeds of change* (209–21). Washington: Smithsonian Institution Press.

Bibliography

Adams, C.F. (ed.). 1876. *Familiar letters of John Adams and his wife Abigail Adams*. New York: Hurd & Houghton.

American Dietetic Association. 1988. *Dietetics in the 21st century: a strategic plan for the American Dietetic Association*. Chicago: American Dietetic Association.

American Restaurant Magazine. 1932. A market analysis of the restaurant industry. Chicago: Peterson.

Armstrong, K. 1988. *Holy war, the Crusades and their impact to today's world*. New York: Anchor Books/Doubleday.

Ashe, T. 1808. *Travels in America in 1806*. London: R. Phillips.

Atwater, W.O. 1887. The chemistry of foods and nutrition. *Century Magazine* 34(1):59–74.

———. 1888a. The pecuniary economy of food. *Century Magazine* 35(3): 437–46.

———. 1888b. What we should eat. *Century Magazine* 36(2):257–64.

Bartlett, R.A. 1989. Donner Pass. *World Book Encyclopedia* 5:311. Chicago: World Book.

Beals, R.L., and H. Hoijer. 1971. *An introduction to anthropology* (4th ed.). New York: Macmillan Company.

Beaver, D. Iron and steel. *World Book Encyclopedia* 10:436–53. Chicago: World Book.

Bernstein, I. 1970. *The lean years*. Baltimore: Penguin.

Black, M. 1992. *The Medieval cookbook*. New York: Thames and Hudson.

Blankenhorn. D. 1978. Progression and regression of femoral atherosclerosis in man. In A.M. Gotto and R. Padetti (eds.), *Atherosclerosis Reviews* 3:169–81. New York: Raven Press.

Boggs, M.M., and C.L. Rasmussen. 1959. Modern food processing. In *Food, the yearbook of agriculture 1959* (418–33). Washington: USDA.

Bolaffi, A., and D. Lulay. 1989. The foodservice industry: continuing into the future with an old friend. *Food Technology* 43(9):258–66.

Bonifay, M.F., and E. Bonifay. 1963. Un gisement à faune épi-villafranchienne à Saint-Estève-Janson (Bouches-du-Rhône). *C.R. Acad. Sci. Paris* 256:1136–38.

Bosley, G.C., and M.G. Hardinge. 1992. Seventh-day Adventists: dietary standards and concerns. *Food Technology* 46(10):112–13.

Bowditch, H.I. 1877. The growth of children. Report of the Massachusetts Board of Health. Cited in R. Cummings, 1970. *The American and his food* (rev.) (89–90). New York: Arno Press.

Bowles, G.T. 1932. *New types of old Americans at Harvard and at eastern women's colleges.* Cambridge: Harvard University Press.

Braidwood, R.J. 1960. The agricultural revolution. *Scientific American* 203:130–48.

Braidwood, R.J., and B. Howe. 1960. *Prehistoric investigations in Iraqi Kurdistan.* Studies in ancient oriental civilization, No. 31. Chicago: University of Chicago Press.

Brayley, A.W. 1909. *Bakers and baking bread in Massachusetts.* Boston: Master Baker's Association of Massachusetts.

Bryant, C.A., A. Courtney, B.A. Markesbery, and K.M. DeWalt. 1985. *The cultural feast.* St. Paul, MN: West Publishing Company.

Burk, M.D. 1961. *Trends and patterns in U.S. food consumption.* USDA Handbook No. 214. Washington: USDA.

Burn, A.R. 1967. *A traveller's history of Greece.* New York: Funk and Wagnalls.

Butrum, R.R., C.K. Clifford, and E. Lanza. 1988. NCI dietary guidelines: rationale. *Am. J. Clin. Nut.* 48(suppl.):882–95.

Butzer, K.W. 1989. Prehistoric people. In *World Book Encyclopedia* 15:748–50. Chicago: World Book.

Campbell, J. 1988. *The power of myth.* New York: Doubleday.

Carcopino, J. 1940. *Daily life in ancient Rome: the people and the city at the height of the Empire.* New Haven, CT: Yale University Press.

Cassidy, C.M. 1980. Nutrition and health in agriculturists and hunter-gatherers. In N.W. Jerome, R.F. Kandel, and G.H. Pelto (eds.), *Nutritional anthropology* (117–45). Pleasantville, NY: Redgrave Publishing Company.

Chaudry, M.M. 1992. Islamic food laws: philosophic basis and practical implications. *Food Technology* 46(10):92–93, 104.

Chitwood, O.P. 1961. *Colonial America.* New York: Harper and Row.

Columbia Broadcasting System. 1969. Hunger in America.

Coon, C.S. 1951. *Cave explorations in Iran, 1949.* Philadelphia: University of Pennsylvania Museum.

———. 1954. *The story of man: from the first human to primitive culture and beyond.* New York: Knopf.

Cooper, T. 1794. *Some information respecting America.* Dublin: William Porter.

Crosby, A.W. 1972. *The Columbian exchange.* Westport, CT: Greenwood Press.

Cummings, R.O. 1970. *The American and his food* (rev.). New York: Arno Press.

Cussler, M., and M. deGive. 1952. *Twixt the cup and the lip.* New York: Twayne.

Dahlberg, F. 1981. Introduction. In F. Dahlberg (ed.), *Woman the gatherer* (1–33). New Haven, CT: Yale University Press.

Darlington, C.D. 1963. *Chromosome botany and the origins of cultivated plants.* New York: Hafner Publishing Company.

Defnet, M.A., J. Ducat, T. Eggericks, and M. Poulain. 1986. *From Grez-Doiceau to Wisconsin.* Bruxelles, Belgium: De Boeck-Wesmael.

Desrosier, N.W. 1963. *Food preservation* (2nd ed.). Westport, CT: Avi Publishing Company.

De Voe, T. 1867. *The market assistant.* New York: Hurd and Houghton.

Dick, E. 1937. *The sod-house frontier, 1854–1900.* New York: D. Appleton-Century Company.

Dobyus, H.F. 1983. *Their number became thinned: Native American population dynamics in eastern North America.* Knoxville: University of Tennessee Press.

Dort, W., and J.K. Jones. 1970. *Pleistocene and recent environments on the Great Plains.* Lawrence: University of Kansas Press.

Douglas, M. 1972. Deciphering a meal. *Daedalus* 101:61–81.

Douglas, P. 1930. *Real wages in the United States, 1890–1926.* Boston: Houghton Mifflin.

Downes, T.W. 1989. Food packaging in the IFT era: five decades of unprecedented growth and change. *Food Technology* 43:228–40.

Dustan, D. 1991. Dinner drinking habits changing. *Green Bay (WI) Press Gazette,* August 1:A-6.

Eaton, S.B., and M.J. Konner. 1985. Stone Age nutrition: implications for today. *Contemporary Nutrition* 10:12.

Eblen, J. 1974. New estimates of the vital rates of the United States black population during the nineteenth century. *Demography* 11(2):301–19.

Eisenberg, J.F. 1981. *The mammalian radiations.* Chicago: University of Chicago Press.

Elson, J. 1992. The millennium of discovery. *Time,* Fall 1992:16–26.

Erdman, J.W., Jr. 1989. Nutrition: past, present, and future. *Food Technology* 43(9):220–27.

Estioko-Griffin, A., and P. Bion Griffin. 1981. Woman the hunter: the Agta. In F. Dahlberg (ed.), *Woman the gatherer* (121–41). New Haven, CT: Yale University Press.

Etherton, T. 1993. The new bio-tech foods. *Food and Nutrition News* 65(3):13–15.

Fearon, H. 1818. *Sketches of America.* London: Longman, Hurst, Rees, Orme, and Brown.

Ferguson, S. 1989. *Soul Food.* New York: Grove Press.

Fogel, R.W., S.L. Engerman, and J. Trussell. 1982. Exploring the uses of data on height. *Social Science History* 6(4):401–21.

Food and Agriculture Organization. 1987. *1948–1985 World crops and livestock statistics.* Rome: United Nations.

———. 1994. World wheat, rice, and corn production, 1990. In *World Almanac* (128). Mahwah, NJ: World Almanac.

Food and Drug Administration. 1990. *Food labeling: mandatory status of nutrition labeling and nutrient content revision.* Fed. Reg. 55:29476–29486. Washington: Food and Drug Administration.

Food Technology. 1992. Food guide pyramid replaces the basic 4 circle. *Food Technology* 46(7):64–65.

Foote, T. 1991. Where Columbus was coming from. *Smithsonian* 22(9):28–41.

Ford, P.L. (ed.). 1894. *The writings of Thomas Jefferson, III.* New York: G.P. Putnam's Sons.

Freedman, A.M., and R. Gibson. 1991. Maker of Simplesse discovers its fake fat elicits thin demand. *Wall Street Journal* July 31:A1, A5.

Gates, W.G., Jr. 1989. Porcelain. *World Book Encyclopedia* 15:678–81. Chicago: World Book.

General Foods Corporation. 1962. *Joys of Jell-O.* White Plains, NY.

Gillett, L.L., and P.B. Rice. 1931. *Influences of education on the food habits of some New York City families.* New York: New York Assoc. for Improving the Condition of the Poor.

Glick, J., and C. Schaefer. 1991. The Columbian exchange. *U.S. News and World Report*, July 8: Special 6-page pullout.

Goldblith, S.A. 1989. Fifty years of progress in food science and technology: from art based on experience to technology based on science. *Food Technology* 43(9):88–107, 286.

———. 1992. The legacy of Columbus, with particular reference to foods. *Food Technology* 46(10):62–85.

Goodrich, S. 1850. *Recollections of a lifetime, I.* New York: Auburn, Miller, Orton and Mulligan.

Gordon, K.E. 1987. Evolutionary perspectives in human diet. In F.E. Johnston (ed.), *Nutritional anthropology* (3–39). New York: Alan R. Liss.

Gotto, A.M. 1979. Is atherosclerosis reversible? *J. Am. Diet. Assoc.*, 74(5): 551–57.

Gould, B. 1869. Investigations in the military and anthropological statistics of American soldiers. New York: United States Sanitary Commission. Cited in R. Cummings, *The American and his food* (rev.). New York: Arno Press.

Graham, E. 1991. McDonald's pickle: he began fast food but gets no credit. *Wall Street Journal*, August 15:A-1, A-10.

Griffin, J.B. 1964. The northeast woodlands area. In J.D. Jennings and E. Norbeck (eds.), *Prehistoric man in the New World* (6th ed.) (223–58). Chicago: University of Chicago Press.

Grover, K. (ed.). 1987. *Dining in America, 1850-1900.* Amherst: University of Massachusetts Press and Rochester, NY: Margaret Woodbury Strong Museum.

Hale, E. 1903. *Memories of a hundred years, I.* New York: Macmillan.

Hall, Richard L. 1989. Pioneers in food science and technology, "giants in the earth." *Food Technology* 43(9):186–95.

Hall, Robert L. 1991. Savoring Africa in the new world. In H.J. Viola and C. Margolis, *Seeds of change* (161–69). Washington: Smithsonian Institution Press.

Hampe, E.C., and M. Wittenberg. 1964. *The lifeline of America—development of the food industry.* New York: McGraw-Hill.

Harlan, J.R. 1976. The plants and animals that nourish man. *Scientific American* 235(3):88–97.

Harlander, S. 1989. Food biotechnology: yesterday, today, and tomorrow. *Food Technology* 43(9):196–206.

Harris, M. 1979. *Cultural materialism: the struggle for a science of culture.* New York: Random House.

———. 1980. *Culture, people, and nature: an introduction to general anthropology* (3rd ed.). New York: Harper and Row.

———. 1987. Foodways: historical overview and theoretical prolegomenon. In M. Harris, and E.B. Ross (eds.), *Food and evolution* (57–90). Philadelphia: Temple University Press.

Harris, M., and E.B. Ross. 1987. Food and evolution. Philadelphia: Temple University Press.

Hawkins, N., and A. Hawkins. 1976. *The American regional cookbook.* Englewood Cliffs, NJ: Prentice Hall.

Hayden, B. 1981a. Research and development in the Stone Age: technological transitions among hunter-gatherers. *Current Anthropology* 22:529–48.

———. 1981b. Subsistence and ecological adaptations of modern hunter-gatherers. In R.S. Harding and G. Teleki (eds.), *Omnivorous primates* (344–421). New York: Columbia University Press.

Hiemstra, S.J. 1968. *Food consumption, prices and expenditures.* U.S. Dept. Agric., Ec. Res. Serv., Agric Rep. 138, Washington, D.C.

Higgs, R. 1975. Mortality in rural America, 1870–1920: estimates and conjectures. *Explorations in Economic History* 10(2):177–95.

Hill, M.M. 1964. Labels on food products. *Nutrition Program News.*

Hill, W.C.O. 1949. Some points in the enteric anatomy of the Great Apes. *Proceedings of the Zoological Society of London* 119:19–32.

Hoebel, E.A., and E. Frost. 1976. *Cultural and social anthropology.* New York: McGraw Hill.

Horn, M., and D. Hawkins. 1991. The Spain that Columbus left behind. *U.S. News and World Report,* July 8:36–37.

Howell, F.C. 1966. Observations on the earlier phases of the European lower paleolithic. *American Anthropologist* 68:88–201.

Institute of Food Technologists. 1989. Top ten food science innovations, 1939–1989. Staff Report. *Food Technology* 43(9):308.

———. 1990. Fat substitute update. *Food Technology* 44(3):92–97.

Jenks, J.W., and W.J. Lauck. 1926. *The immigration problem.* New York: Funk and Wagnall.

Jennings, J.D. 1964. The desert west. In J.D. Jennings and E. Norbeck (eds.), *Prehistoric man in the New World* (6th ed.) (149–74). Chicago: University of Chicago Press.

———. 1968. *Prehistory of North America.* New York: McGraw-Hill.

Jennings, J.D., and E. Norbeck (eds.). 1964. *Prehistoric man in the New World* (6th ed.). Chicago: University of Chicago Press.

Jensen, L.B. 1953. *Man's foods.* Champaign, IL: Garrard Press.

Jernegan, M. 1959. *The American colonies 1492–1750.* New York: Frederick Ungar Publishing Company.

Jerome, N.W. 1972. Individualized home diets: responses to food diversity in an "economically depressed" U.S. urban community. *Federation Proceedings* (Abstracts) 31(2):718.

———. 1979. Changing nutritional styles within the context of the modern family. In D.P. Hynovich and M.U. Barnard (eds.), *Family Health Care* (2nd ed.) (194). New York: McGraw-Hill.

———. 1981. The U.S. dietary pattern from an anthropological perspective. *Food Technology* 35(2): 37–42.

Johnston, F.E. 1982. *Physical anthropology.* Dubuque, IA: Wm. C. Brown Company.

———. (ed.). 1987. *Nutritional anthropology.* New York: Alan R. Liss.

Jones, E. 1990. *American food* (rev.). Woodstock, NY: Overlook Press.

Jones, J. 1985. *Labor of love, labor of sorrow: black women, work, and the family from slavery to the present.* New York: Basic Books.

Joseph, C.C. 1974. Religions of India. In F. Moraes and E. Howe (eds.), *India* (114–25). New York: McGraw Hill.

Kephart, H. 1929. *Our southern highlanders.* New York: Macmillan.

Kessler-Harris, A. 1982. *Out to work.* New York: Oxford University Press.

Kilara, A., and K.K. Iya. 1992. Food and dietary habits of the Hindu. *Food Technology* 46(10): 94–104.

Kirkegaard, P. 1989. Fat substitutes: taste great—less fattening. *Hazelton Food Science Newsletter* 3(31):1. Madison, WI: Hazelton Laboratories America.

Kittler, P., and K. Sucher. 1989. *Food and culture in America.* New York: Van Nostrand Reinhold.

Klein, R.G. 1979. Stone Age exploitation of animals in southern Africa. *American Scientist* 67:151–60.

Kliks, M. 1978. Paleodietetics: a review of dietary fiber in preagricultural human diets. In G.A. Spiller and R.J. Amen (eds.), *Topics in dietary fiber research* (181–202). New York: Plenum Press.

Krieger, A.D. 1964. Early man in the New World. In J.D. Jennings and E. Norbeck (eds.), *Prehistoric man in the New World* (6th ed.) (23–81). Chicago: University of Chicago Press.

La Farge, O. 1956. *A pictorial history of the American Indian.* New York: Crown Publishers.

Lamberg-Karlovsky, C.C., and J.A. Sabloff. 1979. *Ancient civilizations.* Menlo Park, CA: Benjamin Cummings.

Leakey, R.E. 1981. *The making of mankind.* New York: E.P. Dutton.

Leakey, R.E., and R. Lewin. 1977. *Origins.* New York: E.P. Dutton.

Lee, D. 1951. Cultural factors in dietary choice. *Am. J. Clin. Nut.* 5:166.

Lee, R.B. 1968. What hunters do for a living, or how to make out on scarce resources. In R.B. Lee and I. DeVore (eds.), *Man the hunter* (30–48). Chicago: Aldine.

———. 1972. The !Kung bushmen of Botswana. In M.G. Bicchieri (ed.), *Hunters and gatherers today* (1–45). New York: Holt, Rinehart, and Winston.

———. 1979. *The !Kung San.* Cambridge: University Press.

Lee, R.B., and I. DeVore. 1968. *Man the hunter.* Chicago: Aldine.

Leveille, G.A. 1990. Summary of talk "Healthy foods: emerging opportunities for food science and technology," given at the Eighth Annual Midwest Food

Processing Conference, La Crosse, WI, October 2, 1989. In J.D. Dziezak, Midwest processing conference, *Food Technology* 44(4): 56–64.

Levenstein, H.A. 1988. *Revolution at the table.* New York: Oxford University Press.

Levy, A.S., and J.T. Heimbach. 1990. Recent public education efforts about health and diet. In *Conference proceedings of American Council of Consumer Interest.* New Orleans, LA: April.

Liebman, B. 1990. The changing American diet. *Nutrition Action Healthletter* (May 8–9). Washington: Center for Science in the Public Interest.

Lindhert, P.H., and J.G. Williamson. 1976. Three centuries of inequality. In P. Usedling (ed.), *Research in Economic History* 1:69–123.

Lord, L., and S. Burke. 1991. America before Columbus. *U.S. News and World Report,* July 8:36–37.

Lowenberg, M.E., E.N. Todhunter, E.D. Wilson, M.C. Feeney, and J.R. Savage. 1968. *Food and man.* New York: John Wiley and Sons.

Lowenberg, M.E., E.N. Todhunter, E.D. Wilson, J.R. Savage, and J.L. Lubawski. 1979. *Food and people* (3rd ed.). New York: John Wiley and Sons.

Lund, D. 1989. Food processing: from art to engineering. *Food Technology* 43(9): 242–47.

Lusk, G. 1922. A history of metabolism. In L.F. Barker, R.G. Hoskins, and H.O. Mosenthal (eds.), *Endocrinology and metabolism* (3:3–78). New York: D. Appleton and Company.

Lutes, D.T. 1936. *The country kitchen.* Boston: Little, Brown.

Lyman, B. 1989. *A psychology of food.* New York: Van Nostrand Reinhold.

Lynd, R.S., and H. Lynd. 1929. *Middletown, a study in American culture.* New York: Harcourt and Brace.

McCollum, E.V. 1957. *A history of nutrition.* Boston: Houghton Mifflin Company.

McIntosh, E. 1986. Hard food. *Newmonth* 30(8):22–23.

———. 1987. Infant nutrition. *Newmonth* 31(5):23.

McMahon, B. 1974. Infant mortality in the United States. In C.L. Erhardt and J. Berlin (eds.), Mortality and morbidity in the United States (189–209). Cambridge: Harvard University Press.

McMaster, J. 1883. *A history of the United States from the Revolution to the Civil War, I.* New York: D. Appleton & Co.

Martin, E.W. 1942. *The standard of living in 1860.* Chicago: University of Chicago Press.

Martin, J.K. 1989a. Colonial life in America. *World Book Encyclopedia* 4:786–813. Chicago: World Book.

———. 1989b. Revolutionary War in America. *World Book Encyclopedia* 16:274–91. Chicago: World Book.

Martineau, H. 1837. *Society in America, II.* London: Saunders and Otley.

Maslow, A.H. 1970. *Motivation and personality.* New York: Harper and Row.

May, J.M. 1957. The geography of food and cooking. *International Record of Medicine* 170:231.

Mayo Foundation for Medical Education and Research. 1990. Sugar substitutes. *Mayo Clinic Newsletter* August: 3–4.

Mead, M. 1955. *Cultural patterns and technical change. A manual prepared by the World Federation for Mental Health.* New York: New American Library.

Meeker, E. 1972. The improving health of the United States, 1850–1915. *Explorations in Economic History* 9(3):353–73.

Meggitt, M.J. 1962. *Desert people: a study of the Walbiri aborigines of Central America*. Sydney: Angus and Robertson.

Mesick, J.L. 1922. *The English traveller in America, 1785–1835*. New York: Columbia University Press.

Milton, K. 1981. Distribution patterns of tropical plant foods as an evolutionary stimulus to mental development in primates. *American Anthropologist* 83: 534–48.

———. 1987. Primate guts and gut morphology: implications for hominid evolution. In M. Harris and E. Ross (eds.), *Food and evolution* (93–115). Philadelphia: Temple University Press.

Mintz, S. 1991. Pleasure, profit, and satiation. In H.J. Viola and C. Margolis, *Seeds of change* (112–29). Washington: Smithsonian Institution Press.

Morey, D.F. 1994. The early evolution of the domestic dog. *American Scientist* 82(4): 336–47.

Monsen, E.R. 1989. The 1980s: a look at a decade of growth through the pages of the Journal. *J. Am. Diet. Assoc.* 89(12):1742–46.

Morison, S.E. 1965. *The Oxford history of the American people*. New York: Oxford University Press.

———. 1989. Christopher Columbus. In *World Book Encyclopedia* 4:857–58. Chicago: World Book.

Müller-Beck, H. 1967. On migration across the Bering land bridge in the Upper Pleistocene. In D.M. Hopkins (ed.), *The Bering land bridge* (373–408). Stanford, CA: Stanford University Press.

Nash, M. 1963. Burmese Buddhism in everyday life. *American Anthropologist* 65: 285.

National Cancer Institute, Committee on Diet, Nutrition and Cancer. 1982. *Diet, nutrition and cancer*. Washington: National Academy Press.

National Research Council. 1943. *Recommended dietary allowances*. Report of the Food and Nutrition Board, Reprint and Circular Series No. 115, 6 pp. Washington: National Research Council.

———. 1945. *The problem of changing food habits*. Bulletin 111. Washington: National Research Council.

———. 1989. *Recommended dietary allowances* (10th ed.). Washington: National Academy Press.

Nichols, N. 1959. *The country cookbook*. Garden City, NY: Doubleday and Company.

O'Hare, W.P. 1985. *Poverty in America: trends and new patterns*. Population Bulletin 40(3):June. Washington: Population Reference Bureau.

Olmsted, F.L. 1857. *A journey through Texas*. New York: Dix, Edwards and Co.

———. 1860. *A journey in the back country*. New York: Mason Brothers.

O'Neill, C. 1990. Communicating the concepts of good nutrition in the 1990s. *J. Am. Diet. Assoc.* 90(3):373–74.

Osborn, A.J. 1977. Strandloopers, mermaids and other fairy tales: ecological determinants of marine resource utilization. In L.R. Binford (ed.), *For theory building in archaeology: essays on faunal remains, aquatic resources, spatial analysis, and systemic modeling* (157–205). New York: Academic Press.

Owen, Al, and R. Frankle. 1986. *Nutrition in the community.* St. Louis: Times Mirror/Mosby.

Pamela, P. 1969. *Soul food cookbook.* Bergenfield, NJ: New American Library.

Passim, H., and J.W. Bennett. 1943. Social process and dietary change. In *The problem of changing food habits.* National Research Council Bulletin 108. Washington: National Academy of Sciences.

Peckham, G. 1885. Influences of city life on health and development. *Journal of Social Science* 21: 79–89.

Peebles, D.D. 1958. Dried milk product and method of making same. U.S. patent 2,835,586.

Philbeam, D. 1984. The descent of hominoids and hominids. *Scientific American* 250(3): 84–96.

Pike, O.A. 1992. The Church of Jesus Christ of Latter Day Saints: dietary practices and health. *Food Technology* 46(10):118–21.

Putnam, J.J. 1989. *Food consumption, prices and expenditures, 1966–1987.* Stat. Bull. 773. U.S. Dept. Agric., Ec. Res. Serv. Washington: USGPO.

———. 1990. *Food consumption, prices and expenditures, 1967–1988.* Stat. Bull. 804. U.S. Dept. Agric., Ec. Res. Serv. Washington: USGPO.

———. 1991. *Food consumption, 1970–1990.* Food Review 14(3): 2–12.

Rao, S.L.N. 1973. On long-term trends in the United States, 1850–1968. *Demography* 10(3): 405–19.

Reed, C.A. 1977. *Origin of agriculture.* The Hague: Mouton.

Regal, P.S. 1977. Ecology and evolution of flowering plant dominance. *Science* 196: 622–29.

Regenstein, J.M., and C.E. Regenstein. 1979. An introduction to the kosher (dietary) laws for food scientists and food processors. *Food Technology* 33(1): 89–99.

Rice, E. 1973. *The five great religions.* New York: Four Winds Press.

Richardson, B.W. 1887. *The health of nations, a review of the works of Edwin Chadwick,* vol. 2. London: Longmans, Green and Company.

Rischin, M. 1989. Immigration. In *World Book Encyclopedia* 10:82–87. Chicago: World Book.

Robichaux, M. 1989. Boom in fancy coffee pits big marketers, little firms. *Wall Street Journal,* November 6.

Rodman, P.S., and H.M. McHenry. 1980. Bioenergetics and the origins of hominid bipedalism. *American Journal of Physical Anthropology* 52:103–6.

Root, W., and R. de Rochemont. 1976. *Eating in America.* New York: Ecco Press.

Rorabaugh, W.J. 1979. *The alcoholic republic.* New York: Oxford University Press.

Ross, E.B. 1980. Patterns of diet and forces of production: an economic and ecological history of the ascendancy of beef in the United States diet. In E.B. Ross (ed.), *Beyond the myths of culture* (181–225). New York: Academic Press.

Rozin, P. 1982. Human food selection: the interaction of biology, culture and individual experience. In L.M. Barker (ed.), *The psychology of human food selection* (225–54). Westport, CT: Avi.

———. 1987. Psychobiological perspectives on food preferences and avoidances. In M. Harris and E.B. Ross (eds.), *Food and evolution* (181–205). Philadelphia: Temple University Press.

Sacharow, S., and A.L. Brody. 1987. *Packaging: an introduction*. Duluth, MN: Harcourt Brace Jovanovich.

Schaefer, J. 1936. *The social history of American agriculture*. New York: Macmillan.

Schlossberg, K. 1978. Nutrition and government policy in the United States. In B. Wenkoff (ed.), *Nutrition and national policy* (325). Cambridge, MA: MIT Press.

Scrimshaw, N.S., C.E. Taylor, and J.E. Gordon. 1968. *Interactions of nutrition and infection*. WHO Monograph Series No. 57. Geneva: World Health Organization.

Scrimshaw, N., and V. Young. 1980. The requirements of human nutrition. In A.L. Tobias and P.J. Thompson (eds.), *Issues in nutrition for the 1980s* (50–61). Monterey, CA: Wadsworth Health Sciences Division.

Sears, W.H. 1964. The southeastern United States. In J.D. Jennings and E. Norbeck (eds.), *Prehistoric man in the New World* (6th ed.) (251–87). Chicago: University of Chicago Press.

Senate Select Committee on Nutrition and Human Needs. 1968. *Nutrition and human needs, Part I—problems and prospects. Hearings*. 90th Congress, 2nd session, December 17, 18, 19.

———. 1977. *Dietary goals for the United States* (2nd ed.). December. Hearings. Washington: USGPO.

Senauer, B., E. Asp, and J. Kinsey. 1991. *Food trends and the changing consumer*. St. Paul, MN: Eagan Press.

Shields, J.E., and E. Young. 1990. Fat in fast foods—evolving changes. *Nutrition Today* 25(2):32–35.

Simoons, F.J. 1961. *Eat not this flesh*. Madison: University of Wisconsin Press.

Smith, B.D. 1989. Origin of agriculture in eastern North America. *Science* 246: 1566–67.

Smith, B.J., and R.D. Yonkers. 1990. *The importance of cereal to fluid milk consumption*. Marketing Res. Rep. 8, AE&RS 211. University Park: Pennsylvania State University.

Smith, B.J., R.O. Herrman, and R.H. Warland. 1990. *Milk consumption and consumer concerns about fat, cholesterol and calories*. Marketing Res. Rep. 7, AE&RS 210. University Park: Pennsylvania State University.

Sokolov, R. 1981. *The fading feast*. New York: Farrar, Straus, and Giroux.

———. 1991. *Why we eat what we eat*. New York: Summit Books.

Special Supplemental Program for Women, Infants, and Children. 1976. *Federal Register* 1/12, FR Doc. 76–861.

Steinbeck, J. 1939. *The grapes of wrath*. New York: Viking Press.

Steinberg, R. 1970. *Pacific and Southeast Asian cooking*. New York: Time-Life Books.

Tannahill, R. 1973. *Food in history*. New York: Stein and Day.

Thornton, R. 1987. *American Indian holocaust and survival: population history since 1492*. Norman: University of Oklahoma Press.

Toffler, A. 1980. *The third wave*. New York: William Morrow and Company.

Trollope, F. 1832a. *Domestic manners of the Americans, I*. London: Whittaker, Treacher and Company.

————. 1832b. *Domestic manners of the Americans, II*. London: Whittaker, Treacher and Company.

Ubelaker, D.H. 1988. North American Indian population size, A.D. 1500–1985. *Am. J. Phys. Anthro.* 77(3):289–94.

————. 1992. North American Indian population size. In J.W. Verano and D.H. Ubelaker (eds.), *Disease and demography in the Americas* (169–76). Washington: Smithsonian Institution Press.

Underwood, J. 1979. *Human variation and human micro-evolution*. Englewood Cliffs, NJ: Prentice Hall.

United States Bureau of the Census. 1975. *Historical statistics of the U.S., 1914–1936*. Washington: USGPO.

United States Congress, Office of Technology Assessment. 1992. *A new technological era for American agriculture*. OTA-F474. Washington: USGPO.

United States Department of Agriculture. 1943. *National wartime nutrition guide*. Washington: USGPO.

————. 1957. *Dietary levels in households in the United States. Household Food Consumption Survey, 1955*. USDA Report No. 6. Washington: USGPO.

————. 1976. *1961–75 Food Stamp Program*. Food and Nutrition Service, FNS-118 (rev.). Washington: USGPO.

United States Department of Agriculture, Agricultural Research Service. 1958. *Food for fitness—a daily food guide*. Leaflet No. 424. Washington: USGPO.

United States Department of Agriculture, Human Nutrition Information Service. 1989. *Preparing foods and planning menus using the Dietary Guidelines*. Home and Garden Bulletin 232–8:11. Washington: USGPO.

————. 1992. *The food guide pyramid*. Home and Garden Bulletin 252. Washington: USGPO.

United States Department of Agriculture and United States Department of Health and Human Services. 1980. *Nutrition and your health: dietary guidelines for Americans*. Home and Garden Bulletin No. 232. Washington: USGPO.

————. 1990. *Nutrition and your health: dietary guidelines for Americans* (3rd ed.). Home and Garden Bulletin No. 232. Washington: USGPO.

United States Department of Commerce, Bureau of the Census. 1975. *Historical Statistics of the U.S. 1914–1936*. Washington: USGPO.

————. 1976. *Historical statistics of the United States*. Vols. 1 and 2. Washington: USGPO.

United States Department of Health and Human Services, Public Health Service. 1990. *Healthy people 2000. National health promotion and disease prevention objectives*. Washington: USGPO.

United States Department of Health, Education, and Welfare, Food and Drug Administration. 1975. *Read the label, set a better table*. Leaflet. DHEW Pub. No. (FDA)75–4001. Rockville, MD.

United States Fresh Fruit and Vegetable Association. 1988. *The produce industry handbook*. Alexandria, VA: The Association.

Van Doren, C. 1991. *A history of knowledge*. New York: Carol Publishing Group.

Van Leeuwarden, J.H. 1920. Drop a coin and get your pie. *American Restaurant* July: 24.

Van Syckle, C. 1945a. Some pictures of food consumption in the United States: part I, 1630–1860. *J. Am. Diet. Ass.* 19:508–12.

———. 1945b. Some pictures of food consumption in the United States: part II, 1860–1941. *J. Am. Diet. Ass.* 21:690–95.

Vavilov, N.I. 1951. *The origin, variation, immunity and breeding of cultivated plants.* New York: Ronald Press Company.

Verano, J.W., and D.H. Ubelaker. 1991. Health and disease in the pre-Columbian world. In H.J. Viola and C. Margolis (eds.), *Seeds of change* (209–21). Washington: Smithsonian Institution Press.

——— (eds.). 1992. *Disease and demography in the Americas.* Washington: Smithsonian Institution Press.

Viola, H.J. 1991. Seeds of change. In H.J. Viola and C. Margolis (eds.), *Seeds of change* (11–15). Washington: Smithsonian Institution Press.

Volney, C. 1804. *View of the climate and soil of the United States of America.* London: J. Johnson.

Walford, C. 1879. *The famines of the world: past and present.* London: E. Stanford.

Wallingford, J.C. 1994. Nutrition labeling: help or hindrance? *Nutrition and the M.D.* 20(1):1–3.

Wedel, W.R. 1961. *Prehistoric man on the Great Plains.* Norman: University of Oklahoma Press.

———. 1964. The Great Plains. In J.D. Jennings and E. Norbeck (eds.), *Prehistoric man in the New World* (6th ed.) (193–220). Chicago: University of Chicago Press.

Wenkam, N.S. 1969. Cultural determinants of nutritional behavior. *Nutrition Program News.* July/August.

White, E.G. 1905. *The ministry of healing.* Mountain View, CA: Pacific Press Publishing Association.

———. 1938. *Counsels on diet and foods.* Washington, DC: Review and Herald Publishing Company.

White, L. 1962. *Medieval technology and social changes.* London: Oxford University Press.

White House Conference on Food, Nutrition, and Health. 1970. *Final report.* Washington: USGPO.

Williams, S. 1985. *Savory suppers and fashionable feasts: dining in Victorian America.* New York: Pantheon.

Williams, S.R. 1989. *Nutrition and diet therapy* (6th ed.). St. Louis: Times Mirror/Mosby College Publishing.

Woodburne, J. 1968. An introduction to Hazda ecology. In R.B. Lee and I. DeVore (eds.), *Man the hunter* (49–55). Chicago: Aldine.

World Almanac. *1994.* Mahwah, NJ: World Almanac.

Wyse, R.D. 1989. Sugar. *World Book Encyclopedia* 18:959–61. Chicago: World Book.

Yesner, D.R. 1987. Life in the "Garden of Eden": causes and consequences of the adopting of marine diets by human societies. In M. Harris and E.B. Ross (eds.), *Food and evolution* (285–310). Philadelphia: Temple University Press.

Zeuner, F.E. 1963. *A history of domesticated animals.* London: Hutchinson and Company.

Index

About the Author

ELAINE N. McINTOSH, Ph.D., R.D., is Professor Emerita of Human Biology at the University of Wisconsin, Green Bay. She is coauthor, with Elizabeth Green, of *On Your Own in the Kitchen* (1985), a cooking guide for nonreaders based on sound nutritional principles. She has contributed chapters to internationally published books and government publications in addition to numerous articles in reputable scientific journals of all kinds since 1954. She has been a long-time nutritional and health writer for *Newmonth*.